# DON'T WORRY. BE HEALTHY!

*HOW TO AVOID*

*OBSESSING ABOUT YOUR HEALTH*

## BY MARTIN P. SOLOMON, MD

Ansco Publishing
Box 959
Brookline, Mass 02446


Library of Congress Catalog Card Number
99-94524


ISBN 0-9671145-0-0


Cover design and illustration by Rachel Simon

# ACKNOWLEDGEMENTS

This project would not have been possible without the support, encouragement and editorial input of my wife. Her strength and courage through her illness and treatment served as my inspiration to persevere with my writing. The hours of typing and creating I stole from her at the end of my long day at work and on vacations were given without question and for this I am grateful. Betsy, where would I be without you?

The creative drive and appreciation for the written word are the gift of my mother who enticed me with books from my early childhood. When I was just a goof-off in the sixth grade, she refused to accept my apparent limitations. Thank you for seeing more in me and gently pushing me along.

My father taught me to see every day as a new opportunity. His indomitable optimism and appreciation for life exuded a spirituality that has kept me on the right path.

My father-in-law served as my guide and mentor and taught me self-discipline, without which I could never have completed this work. My mother-in-law opened her home and provided much of the time and rest I needed to concentrate on this project.

Lesley, Lori and Amy, my three daughters, provided editorial and grammatical review and an unbiased belief in the importance of my writing.

Lewis Cohen, my brother-in-law, provided essential business guidance.

In the nascent phases of this book, Peter Davison provided encouragement and advice that helped to launch the work. His medical visits to me often ended in discussions about the proper approach to my efforts. Josephine Simon guided me through the morass of the creative and business aspects of book preparation. She urged me onward when my spirit flagged.

Walter and Sue Cahners deserve special thanks for their extensive editorial review and insightful suggestions.

Many others helped with editorial review and criticism including Jonathan Wilson, Ina Yaloff, Alan Feldman, Dr. Joseph Sequeira,

## Acknowledgements

Michael and Lynn Hess, My son-in-law Geoffrey Hess and soon to be son-in-law Michael York, Dr. Fred Bierman, Rachel Simon and her parents Toby and Cantor Murray Simon, my partner Dr. Jeffrey Bass, Ken Shulman, Sandy Krakoff and my office manager and friend Amy Goldman. I particulary want to thank Tod Herzog for his help in choosing a title.

My thanks go to Joel Skolnick at The PrintCentre for expeditious copying and production assistance and to my good friend and attorney Martin Shulkin for his expert legal counsel.

# TABLE OF CONTENTS

*This work is dedicated to my patients past and present in appreciation for placing their trust in me, for allowing me into their lives and for enabling me to learn from them.*

*It is particularly dedicated to Rachel Simon, dear friend and patient, whose creative effort produced the design and artwork on the cover of this book.*

# *1*

## THE UNFORGIVING MINUTE

The most important lesson I learned about how to live well was taught to me by my grandfather and my wife's grandfather, two hard working simple men with old country values. They both told me at different times that living a good life had to do with being proud of who you are and what you have done. Looking back on more than 90 years of living, they both told me that in the end, all you have to leave behind of real value is a good name. Material possessions can vanish overnight and often do. Fortunes and business success stored away over decades are evanescent. Few people will remember that you were tall or short, fat or thin, wrinkled or smooth of face. But most will remember if you lived a good life or wasted it away, if you gave to your community, if you were a good parent who raised children to be proud of, if you were a good friend or helped lost souls find their way. Few will remember that you were in good shape or that you looked trim in your clothes. Instead, they will recall "She was always tired and complained a lot" or "she was always upbeat and could cheer up a dismal day."

People who see beyond themselves to the community around them, often overcome personal handicaps of size, speech, vision, hearing, and mobility and recognize that this is an imperfect world. There is so much to do to make it right and so little time to waste on complaining or worrying about things you can't change. They strive to "fill the unforgiving minute with sixty seconds worth of distance run..." On the other hand, many people today seem to be surrounded by a reflective cloud that interprets all worldly events and calamities through the impact on themselves. If it's too cold, it will make their arthritis hurt. If a friend gets cancer, they worry that they are next. If they develop an illness, whether trivial or grave, it is perceived as the end of the natural world. They will devote endless hours worrying and visiting all forms of physicians, osteopaths, chiropractors and acupuncturists.

In the course of my daily visits with patients over a period of more than 20 years I have observed a gradual change in the intensity of concern people display about their potential for acquiring some dreadful illness or for dealing with the end of life. As our population ages and the density of our civilization increases, we become painfully aware of illness in our friends, neighbors and family. We sense and fear our own mortality. While it is a truism that we will all develop some terminal problem sometime in our lives, that being the nature of life, most of us are healthy most of the time. I don't deny that many of us will develop upper respiratory virus colds, headaches from stress or being overtired, backaches from straining or lifting, sore muscles and joints from work or exercise, and upset gastrointestinal tracts from eating the wrong food at the wrong time or as the natural result of aging. However, these are usually self-limited problems and, in most cases, will resolve without medical attention. In the vast majority of cases, they are not a sign of some underlying constitutional weakness or lurking disease. They should not be seen as harbingers of death. Studies have demonstrated that most visits to a physician's office and as a result, much of the medical testing that follows is unnecessary.

In spite of this, a large portion of our national budget now goes to paying for what is euphemistically called health care. We are urged by the advertising industry to pursue unhealthy life styles through the use of tobacco, alcohol, rich foods and activities associated with high risk. Simultaneously we are encouraged by the health care industry, often represented by the same advertising firms, to watch for the latest discoveries and technological advances which might prolong our lives and avoid suffering and death. Most magazines, newspapers, and the broadcast media have a special section dedicated to telling us about what's new and hot, often before physicians and the rest of the scientific community have a chance to consider and critically review them. In the current competitive climate, medical institutions fight for a greater share of patient care. Hospitals and ambulatory medical centers promise that they can deliver best the latest and most up to date treatment in the hope of luring substantial numbers of patients into their fold to increase the numbers of covered lives.

We in the medical industry have fostered a climate of obsessive concern about health, illness, suffering and insurability which preys on our cultural focus on youth and immortality. Having people worry about illness and medical problems is good business. Aging is not an acceptable option. We can lift and tuck, suction and trim. We can transplant hair where it has long since left and augment various parts of our anatomy to restore the appearance of youth or even create it where it never existed. Genetic scientists promise to find methods to actually stop aging. The question we encourage our patients to focus on is how to stay young, not how to live well. Advertisers for medical treatments of all sorts are fond of using the saying "If you've got your health, then you've got everything." This is a simple bald-faced lie. You can have good health and still have an empty life. More importantly, you can have less than perfect health and yet feel wonderfully fulfilled.

I recall one patient, a professor at a local college who has been blind since a tumor was removed from behind his eye many years earlier. In spite of his significant handicap, he is happy and successful in his work. He is married to a wonderful and supportive woman and he finds constant reasons to feel positive and upbeat. He loves to teach and his courses are highly sought by students. When I walk out to the waiting room to greet him, he always responds with a ready smile as his wife guides him down the corridor to my office. Once seated, he immediately asks about my health and my family. We spend a significant part of his rare visits to me telling jokes and stories, and our conversation is frequently interrupted with laughter. The medical exam that follows is almost an afterthought. Not only does he feel well, he makes me feel good.

Many more patients continue to come in to see me with complaints focused around their fear of developing the latest disease about which they have read or their friend, neighbor or relative may have acquired. They present with a near mortal fear that a bodily sensation, real or imagined, is a sign of their impending doom or their imminent loss of youth. Regardless of the symptom, the subliminal concern is their potential to develop an illness that will lead to pain and suffering and ultimate shortening of their natural lives. This is perfectly normal and some patients will accept my reassurance as to the benign nature of their malady. An increasing proportion, however, remain fearful and continue to harbor anxieties that cannot be assuaged by a simple office visit. Driven by the media, pharmaceutical manufacturers and the medical profession, they are urged to keep looking for a perfect, simple cure, free of side effects, or that rare and awful diagnosis that they fear will be found if only sufficient scientific testing is applied to the search. The growing prevalence of this misguided public perception of the interaction between scientific research and quality of life is dangerous and counterproductive and leads to new health risks. Rather than enjoy life, we as a culture worry constantly about health and illness. Though many suffer from serious diseases, most of us do not.

I have often wanted to recommend the words of Dr. Seuss in Did I Ever Tell You How Lucky You Are? to my patients with this limited view of their lives and their health. In his wonderfully insightful way, Dr. Seuss reminds us of all the many good fortunes that make life worthwhile. He points out the often forgotten truth that no matter how bad you think things are, somebody is always worse off. One of the great advantages and disadvantages of my job results from seeing people in the worst of life's predicaments—cancer, leukemia, heart disease, AIDS, domestic violence, behavioral and marital problems and depression to name only a painful few. It all sounds rather unpleasant. Patients and friends will often ask me, "How can you deal with this and keep your sanity?" I explain that the experience of helping others to cope with suffering allows me to appreciate my good fortune. Once, as a child I had complained to my mother enviously about a friend with a big house and a fancy car. Why, I asked should we not also have a nicer car and a bigger house? She referred me to a saying that I have never forgotten and which is now a staple of my daily work. "I complained that I had no shoes until I met a man who had no feet." Instead of obsessing about my own discomfort, real or imagined, I was urged to look to the suffering of others, to reach out to help them rather than focus on my own needs. I have never forgotten that simple message.

What has all this got to do with obesity, exercise, fatigue, getting colds, dealing with aches and pains and growing old? Very simply, if you're worried about your brother and sister, your neighbor and your community, the environment and the integrity of the world around you, then there is little time to obsess about issues that will have no impact on your greater goals. You have the sniffles and everybody around you is suffering from the same. It's just a cold. Forget about it. You lifted a sofa and now your back hurts. What did you expect? It will probably hurt for a while and then get better. Forget about it. You still can't get into that outfit you've wanted because you just can't make the changes you need in your schedule and your diet. Forget about it. Accept yourself as you are and begin to deal with the world that is beyond your personal space.

In my own family over the past four years I have watched the development of heart disease and cancer in three of the people who have meant the most to me. My father, a man I loved and admired as much as a son is able, developed lymphoma, fought a valiant battle for seven years and died at home. Each time he went for chemotherapy as he did many times over the course of his illness, he never showed up at the oncology unit without a box of candy for the nurses and receptionists. He worried more about the impact of his illness on others than on himself. As he lay dying in his last week, he would spruce himself up and put on his best smile for my wife who was in an earlier stage of the same illness, lest she suffer from seeing his discomfort. My father-in-law, a man who was both my friend and mentor, developed first heart disease and then one year later lung cancer and then died after a determined two year fight. To the very end he worried as to whether he had done enough to help repair the world. His only regret was that he wished he had more time to accomplish the many goals he had set for himself to try to make the world better for those who followed in his footsteps. At the same time, my wife, the source of all strength and peace in my life, a pillar of health and fitness, developed lymphoma. She has taught me that life is too precious to waste worrying about trivialities. Problems that seemed before to be so important and consuming that we would sit up all night obsessing over them became insignificant when faced with the risk of losing everything.

As I watched each one of them individually and collectively deal with their illnesses and studied my own reactions to the inevitable changes, I developed a new understanding of my patients, their problems and my attitudes towards them. This experience and the deeper understanding it has given me about those issues in life which are really important has driven my desire to write this book.

While every family has illness, as a nation we are the worried well. I have seen hundreds of patients who find their bodily symptoms as their major focus in life and watched this obsession lead to the neglect of their family, their work and their general happiness. Countless patients, unwilling to accept a diagnosis of medically good health, spend hours each day obsessing about their bodily functions and real or perceived malfunctions while missing out on the true joys of living in the real world. To physicians trying to prevent, diagnose and treat disease, the needless distraction created by the public's health obsession can be, at the very least, a source of tremendous frustration. To the healthy but worried well, this excessive focus on illness robs them of precious moments which could be spent enjoying a sunrise or sunset, a cool breeze, the sound of wind blowing through the trees or a child's laughter. This book addresses the major areas of these obsessions and tries to provide some guidance to empower us all to relax, stop worrying and be happy.

# 2

## IF YOU'VE GOT YOUR HEALTH

At 89 years of age, Mrs. Sterling was a remarkable individual. She had outlived two husbands and still maintained an active social schedule, attending local senior citizen events and concerts and traveling with Golden Age groups. I looked forward to her visits to my office, particularly because of the delicious chocolate chip cookies neatly wrapped in paper and tied with a red bow she always brought for me. She would always start off by asking about each of my children and inquiring after the health of my wife and parents, then regale me with stories of the triumphs and tragedies of her children and grandchildren . This year, however, her usual good cheer was interrupted by an air of tension. She did not joke about the crowded waiting room or have any of her usual bounce and confidence. The change in her attitude was striking. I told her it was apparent to me that she had something on her mind. With some initial hesitation, she began to tell me of the recent death of her oldest friend, and for the first time since I had been her doctor, she cried during the visit.

It was a painful moment for both of us. I said, "You must have been very close." She took a deep breath and sighed. Then she began to express concern about some of her own symptoms. The list was long and not in any consistent pattern. Headaches, nausea, gas, aching, fatigue, sleeplessness. She was upset that I had not taken these complaints seriously and had not sent her for a CAT scan of her head, gastrointestinal x-rays or tried new medications as her friends had received. She could have gone on for a while. I asked her to stop for a moment. "What are you really worried about? What are you afraid of?" A long pause followed. Her response was one I have heard thousands of times over the past 20 years, but never from her. "It's no good to be old. You do everything, well, almost everything right. You eat well, look after yourself, stay away from bad things like drugs and whiskey and the wild life, and where do you end up? Old and sick and alone, that's where." I asked her to tell me more about her friend who had died. It was a relationship that spanned a period of more than 75 years from the time they met as young teen-agers. They had experienced all of life's major events together: court-ship, marriages, divorces, careers, illness, children, and grandchil-dren. Their hopes and dreams were always shared and they sup-ported each other during crises. Parts of the story caused her to cry a little more, but some caused her to openly giggle like an adolescent. I told her how fortunate she was to have had such a relationship for so many years, but she already knew that. She needed to be brought back to these good memories.

We sat for a few moments while she regained her composure, then moved to the examination room where I checked carefully for any signs of serious medical problems that might need attention. Aside from a few simple issues which could be dealt with quite easily, she looked reasonably well for her advanced years. When she returned to my office after dressing and having her blood drawn, I reviewed the findings of the examination and told her she appeared to be well. I asked about her plans for the coming year and she told me about her granddaughter's impending marriage, at which point some of the sparkle returned to her now drier eyes. How remarkable, I pointed out, to have so much good fortune and excitement in one lifetime. Though being old was a source of distress for many, and the "Golden Years" might not seem so golden to her now, I suggested that the journey was well worth it. A broad smile appeared, and she clearly relaxed from some of her initial tension. She told me she really had no regrets about her life, though she wasn't quite ready for it to be over, and still had a lot of plans.

I told her I could order the tests she wanted, though I didn't be-lieve they were necessary and I could prescribe some pills for her symptoms, but I thought the side effects would be worse than the problems. She agreed. "I'm probably just tired and stressed. I don't need any medication." We chatted a little more and completed some of the formalities of the usual medical visit, refilling prescriptions and scheduling next year's appointment. Before she left the office, she promised to bring cookies some time in the next week.

Later on the same day, Mark, a young man of 39 came in for his physical examination. He also was in perfect health with no complaints and no risk factors for serious diseases. A detailed review of his bodily systems failed to reveal any evidence of problems and his physical examination was perfect. He was puzzled why I did not feel it necessary to perform a cardiac stress test, a prostate antigen test and a chest x-ray as part of his routine visit. We talked at length about the arguments against using these as well as other tests as screening procedures and then addressed the reasons that made him at his very peak of fitness and productivity, so concerned about health issues.

It became clear that the impact on him of a recent cancer diagnosis in a close friend and the media barrage over new genetic screening tests had him on edge. He worried about his own mortality and the potential effect illness might have on his rising career, his family responsibilities and his dreams for the future. What, he questioned, could he do to be sure he would minimize the risk of illness and disability? How could he be sure he was doing everything possible to keep himself functioning at his peak for an indefinite period? He wanted to be certain he could prevent one of these catastrophes from befalling him. Everywhere he turned he was told to take vitamins, garlic, algae, zinc, low fat-no fat food, exercise like mad, avoid the sun, avoid food additives, stay away from this or that and basically concentrate on keeping his body protected from the dangers of the world around him.

My response was simple and direct:

You take care of yourself. You eat well, exercise regularly, avoid excess alcohol and you don't smoke. You seem, at least until these concerns became an issue, to be happy about your life. You have a normal physical examination. Assuming your blood tests confirm my observations, it is safe to say that you are indeed in good health. Many of the things about which you despair cannot be predicted with enough accuracy to justify all the testing which might be necessary to reassure you. STOP WORRYING ABOUT YOUR HEALTH!

The contrast between these two approaches to life is a striking but typical example of the change I have seen in our national attitude towards the importance of health and illness prevention. While Mrs. Sterling and many of her generation understand their place in the natural order of life, the latter quarter of the twentieth century has seen a change in our focus to the "now". The past is done and the future is unknown. We need to have immediate and total explanation, a sense of certainty about what is and is yet to be. Mark wants a guarantee of good health. He is preoccupied with his fear that in spite of all his efforts to do everything right to maintain his health, all will be taken away if he misses a possible diagnosis of incipient illness. If he had any doubts about this risk, they are certainly diminished by everything he reads in the newspapers or sees on television. He is urged to watch for danger signs of unusual illnesses, have his genetic markers checked, watch out for diseases for which there is new miraculous treatment and yet is found only in a small percentage of the population. He is told to be wary of symptoms that may seem routine but imply an illness which could go unrecognized. In short, he is told not to slip into the complacent feeling that he is well even though he may feel just fine. Danger could be lurking around the corner.

Every day I see people who worry that they are not doing enough to prevent illness. Even among those who are doing very little to maintain their health, the fear of unexpected catastrophe and the need for new diagnostic technology is obvious. Like Mark, they appear to have an insatiable desire for certainty that all is well. This desire for answers changes us all from being people who are occasionally inconvenienced or set upon by illness into a nation of patients and health care consumers. In response to this demand, the health care industry supplies us with a diet of miracle cures, technological advances and mystical alternatives all aimed at nourishing this preoccupation. When a laboratory finds a new potential clue to a scientific mystery or a clinical study reveals new data regarding treatment, its public relations department sends out a press release and plays the latest "discovery" as front page news. If a piece of information suggests a possible link between some herbal or nutritional supplement and some aspect of bodily function, the organic and so-called naturopathic industry whips into action with a proliferation of periodicals as well as promotions for the substance.

When melatonin, a natural occurring substance, was found to be effective and safe for inducing sleep for some people, the so-called health food industry filled the shelves with all sorts of melatonin preparations. Within weeks, various manufacturers were touting the quality of their particular formulation. Patients would call me or write asking if I thought this would help with their sleep problems. They sent promotional material they found in health food stores or articles from newspapers or periodicals of various sorts. The articles and ads were sometimes interesting, more often inappropriately over-exuberant in their remarks, and occasionally down right preposterous. A quick perusal of some of these items could be a terrific source of laughter if they were not taken seriously by so many people. They suggested all sorts of miraculous events which might occur if only their specific brand were used.

In the case of melatonin, I try to explain to my patients that this medication will help with restoring sleep patterns in approximately a third of the those who try it. For those individuals this would be a great medicine for sleep, since it appears to be reasonably safe. For the rest, however, there is currently very little firm evidence that melatonin will change anything in spite of some interesting studies on the effect of melatonin on the immune system. Manufacturers and purveyors present claims about it's benefit in prolonging life, improving immunity, promoting hair growth, and improving sexual function, among other potential benefits. One can easily understand the appeal of such promises. The motives in this process have more to do with personal and corporate profits than with the well being of the general public.

The beta-carotene story is another good example. In the long process of trying to understand why some people get cancer or heart disease and others not, much attention has been focused on food. A popular maxim of the 1960's stated that you are what you eat. Gradually the American public has begun to think a little more carefully about what goes into our collective mouths and bodies. Investigators found that a number of food substances had the ability to protect important structures and chemicals in the body from the destructive action of an important chemical process called oxidation. Many of the toxins which were found to be bad for our health appear to exert some of their most damaging effects by oxidizing body substances. Based on this work, it was logical to conclude that if we ate food containing something that would block this oxidation, i.e. antioxidants, this diet would be good for our health.. Studies demonstrated that antioxidants could indeed reduce the risk of heart disease and cancer. In some cases, such as cancer of the oropharynx (tongue, sinuses and throat), the benefit was striking.

This information was seized upon by all of the health industry. Newspapers, TV health shows, medical newsletters, and talk shows all began to run stories on this simple miracle substance. Many physicians, not wanting to seem ill informed, encouraged their patients to take betacarotene. They often began taking it themselves or were pushed to do so by their spouses. The pharmaceutical industry began pumping out betacarotene pills by the billions and marketing new vitamins with this substance and other antioxidants included. If you weren't taking betacarotene it was hard to keep your head high at the health food store. Large posters extolled the benefit of this or that "natural" brand of betacarotene. Patients came in to see me proud of the size of the doses they were able to consume. Millions of dollars were spent on producing and promoting betacarotene pills. Little mention was made of the fact that a diet high in fresh vegetables would provide all the betacarotene anybody would need.

Just as the betacarotene craze seemed to reach messianic levels, new clinical research revealed problems with consuming regular doses of this substance above the normal dietary level. In fact, the daily consumption of betacarotene may have significantly adverse side effects. For example, excessive amounts can lead to skin changes and liver injury. In addition, regular consumption of extra betacarotene can actually increase the risk of cancer in some people who take it to protect themselves from smoking and other destructive personal habits. This miracle substance which the health industry so vigorously promoted may actually be bad for some. One patient came in recently to tell me about a letter he received from a famous cardiologist at a major Boston teaching hospital. This medical specialist, widely respected by his peers, had been recommending betacarotene from the beginning of the excitement about it's potential value. This patient was surprised at how strongly the letter urged him to stop taking betacarotene and finished with the hope that the patient had not invested heavily in companies producing the substance. The end result of this cycle is typical. Some people made lots of money, the public spent lots of money, and it is unlikely that many ended up healthier.

The enormous industry which involves academia and the business community are the major beneficiaries of all the publicity. In a manner similar to the example cited above, universities are anxious to promote their research and their faculty's discoveries to facilitate fund raising and grant procurement, to say nothing of elevating their image within the academic community. Scientific discoveries attract donors who contribute and graduate students who pay tuition. The business world wants to attract investors and profit from potential opportunities. Witness the sudden explosion of biotechnology stocks once word is leaked to the investing public about a potential treatment. The media wants to sell newspapers, gain viewers or listeners, or attract advertising. Medical professionals and alternative medicine providers benefit by attracting patients to pursue new high cost treatments, tests and procedures to feed their substantial egos and fill their wallets. People worry more about their health, and yet are no healthier.

The public is a receptive audience to this self-promotion. And why shouldn't we be excited about these purported medical breakthroughs? Science, industry and the media pitch their stories to the natural desire to avoid pain, illness and death. Why, we ask, if they can put a man on the moon, can't they find a cure for cancer, AIDS, heart disease, obesity and all the other problems that plague humanity? Turn on the evening news any night and watch Healthwatch, Healthbeat, Medicalwatch or a similar mutation. These shows provide an instant distillation of articles from prestigious medical journals or a public relations blitz from one lab or another anxious to bring attention to their latest work, usually before your doctor has a chance to hear the news. For many, the Wall Street Journal has become the most up to date source of medical news. Most of these medical news flashes have not been subjected to critical review in the medical and scientific community.

It is disingenuous for all parties involved to claim that the motive for promulgating this new information is based on a desire to get essential and critical news to the wider community. We are led to believe that this new information will significantly change our quality of life if we will only subscribe to a steady supply of new therapies, medications and surgical treatments which will ostensibly correct the backward and outdated approaches of the past. The past, of course, ages quickly and includes every moment up to this new discovery.

Often, my wife will call me in my office at 7 am just before I start seeing patients to warn me of something she read in The Boston Globe or heard on the Today Show or Good Morning America. A health reporter will present some new medication or treatment or new research about a treatment currently in use. I know I will receive dozens of phone calls and faxes from anxious patients before the morning is over. First, I warn Amy Goldman, my office manager, so she can prepare the receptionists with a standard response. However, the more persistent or astute patients will get through. To them, I simply say, "Don't get excited. Let me have a chance to review this and if there is anything important, I will get back to you." I also suggest that they shut the sound off the TV when the medical news comes on and avoid reading health sections in the news since they can cause unnecessary alarm. I sometimes wonder if they should include a warning before the health bullets. It should read something like "Warning: The following health news may be irrelevant and unproved. Action taken on the basis of what you are about to hear or read may be dangerous to your physical and mental health."

The debate surrounding screening mammograms is a telling tale. As mammograms became more sensitive over the last decade, breast cancers were found progressively earlier. Physicians continued to recommend annual mammograms after age 40 until a potentially flawed study out of Canada demonstrated no significant benefit from mammograms between ages 40 and 50. Medical organizations and societies were cowed into recommending studies every other year by insurance companies and the federal government who jumped at this opportunity to reduce costs. Suddenly, women were not allowed by their insurance company to have more than five mammograms in this 10 year block. Everybody but the bean counters were uncomfortable with this. We had a suspicion there was something wrong. It seemed that more and more women in their 40's were presenting with advanced breast cancer. Proponents of every other year testing claimed that this was due to finding cancers earlier but not helping survival. Then in 1997 new evidence was published supporting the use of annual mammograms during the fifth decade, leading to a shift in approach again and a backing down of the payers for health care to permit annual screening. It becomes difficult to discern which approach is right, but it should be easy to see that the insurance industry, government spokespersons and others who ran too quickly to change because of new evidence from a few studies were wrong.

Reasonable scientists and physicians recognize the uncertain and tenuous nature of these hectic discoveries. Today's dogma is tomorrow's anathema. I vividly remember as a medical student thirty years ago, listening to the chief of rheumatology describe with disdain the risky practice of community doctors who used cortisone to treat rheumatoid arthritis. These simple non-scientific community doctors used potentially risky treatment to allow their patients to live comfortably. While they were perhaps not totally cognizant of all the potential side effects of the medication, at least they knew their patients felt better. My professor in the academic tower taught us to be more cautious about using such powerful drugs for what was viewed as a chronic illness of living. Today cortisone, along with other powerful medications, has become a mainstay of treatment for advanced forms of this disease by specialists in the field. If those community doctors of 30 years ago were still around, I'm sure they would relish the vindication. The lesson for me, however, is that in medicine there are few absolute truths. The more we learn, the more we realize we don't understand.

In spite of this transitory and evolutionary character of medical and scientific knowledge, the public optimistically listens for each new "discovery", hoping that at any moment some research scientist will find some potion to take care of illness or pain, restore energy to a tired and stressed body, restore vigor and vibrancy. Hence, the proliferation of health newsletters and health fairs run by hospitals, insurance companies and medical groups. An enormous conflict of interest exists in the fact that most of these are underwritten by pharmaceutical manufacturers, insurers and large health care providing organizations. While much good can be achieved by screening for known examples of medical disorders, economic forces all stand to gain financially by encouraging the public to look for new unrecognized cases of disease. Doctors get more patients, hospitals get to perform more tests and use their expensive technology and insurance companies get more customers. Once again we turn people into patients.

This is not to say that the health care industry encourages illness. There is more than enough to go around already. I have heard some of the more paranoid members of our community suggest that many diseases, like AIDS or hypertension, represent a plot by the medical profession to discriminate against politically unpopular groups or just to keep patients flowing into offices, clinics and hospitals. Andrew is a gay hair dresser and old friend and patient in exceptionally good health. As more and more of his friends succumbed to AIDS he became focused on literature suggesting that the virus was planted by Washington politicians and members of the medical profession as a way of destroying the gay community. He would bring me books and pamphlets supporting this position. I tried to point out that this was an exercise in fear and anxiety. There is no such cabal. Modern medicine has no need to make people sick. On the contrary, as the result of many advances in medicine, most people are living longer and more productive lives and go on being cared for by well trained and talented physicians and nurses for years and years.

Unfortunately, a lot of useless care and questionable treatment is imposed on the public by other parts of the health industry that builds profit centers around each new advance. As an illustration, a quick check around the major teaching hospitals will reveal the presence of cardiac risk clinics. These centers were created to meet the demand from people like Mark, our anxious 39 year old, for control of cholesterol and prolongation of life through the use of various interventions such as medication, exercise and diet counseling. In concert with the pharmaceutical industry which actively supports the physicians and hospitals running these units, the health industry once again has tapped into a new source of income.

Rather than send people to their primary care physician who is trained to address the problems of cholesterol and life style changes, patients are encouraged to participate in this costly and medically intensive approach to a potential problem. Yet there is no evidence that it will lead to a prolonged or improved life. At the same time, by plugging people into clinics identified with illness, we turn healthy individuals who thought they were doing OK into patients with illness as part of their identity. I have many patients who insist on seeing a cardiologist every year even though they have no evidence of heart disease. "Just in case", they say, as if by seeing a heart specialist they will be protected from catastrophic heart disease. I usually ask these people, only half in jest, whether they have the plumber and electrician check there home each year, "just in case" there should be a clogged pipe or a short circuit. When it comes to health and illness, clearly many of us are so anxious we will go to any length to get reassurance. We are whipped into a state of fear by the medical profession, the supporting (or parasitizing) industries and the media.

Obesity, back pain, smoking, headaches, heart disease, cancer, ulcers, hypertension represent only a small fraction of the curses for which all would like to find a simple solution. We want a pill, a painless risk free operation, a genetic maneuver or some simple herbal nostrum to cure us. We want to enjoy life, prosper and achieve happiness without having to deal with disease, so we worry about whether or not we are doing the right thing. Should we eat more pasta, protein, complex carbohydrates or more vegetables? Exercise more or less and how? Should we have our skin checked by a skin specialist and how often? The painful truth is that life is imperfect. While for most Americans it might not be nasty, brutish and short, it is inevitably filled with discomforts, maladies and disorders. Most of these, however, will go away on their own like a passing storm. Some will require limited medical attention. Other problems may become more serious and lead to a real life change. Under no circumstance does this mean we need to see ourselves as different people.

I have learned much about this from dealing with people with long-term disabilities such as blindness, hearing impairment, spinal cord disease and crippling forms of cerebral palsy. These people will often come in only once a year for their checkups and will sit in my office cheerfully telling me how well they feel. Like Mrs. Sterling, my 89 year old cookie baker, they view life's cup as half full rather than half empty.

One particular man stands out for me as an example of what we should aspire to and what we need to avoid in our response to illness. Paul is a 38 year old investment advisor with a wonderful wife and two great kids. I look forward to his visits because he is always in such an upbeat and cheerful mood. We often exchange stories about work and family changes. What makes our interaction unusual is that Paul has been unable to hear since birth. We communicate through the minimal amount of signing I have picked up, his ability to read lips and by writing notes. He will occasionally bring a translator along for the visit. When we need to communicate during non-office hours he uses a service provided by the phone company or we talk via e-mail on the internet.

The important message is that Paul doesn't allow his problem to interfere with his ability to enjoy life. He is not a hearing impaired person. He is a father, financial advisor, husband and friend who happens also to be unable to hear. Contrast this with the patient who comes with some minor decrease in hearing from a recent cold, in spite of my reassurances on the phone that this will go away on its own in time. Some will return to see me two or three times and ultimately insist on seeing a hearing specialist for a problem that is clearly self-limited. Their transient hearing problem becomes a medical crisis in their minds. Instead of being people inconvenienced by a cold and it's complications, they become patients suffering from an illness which requires the full efforts of the medical profession to resolve.

Or take the example of Nancy, a 50 year old woman whom I have known since childhood because of our mothers' friendship. Nancy was disabled by cerebral palsy at birth and suffered severe deformities of her arms and legs. With her parents' support she managed to overcome the continuous difficulties of dressing, walking, going to school and just getting around. She is actively employed and exudes an aura of good cheer and friendship to any willing recipient. Juxtapose her visit to me for her once a year routine checkup with the high-powered young business woman who twisted her ankle running a few weeks ago. In spite of the natural healing which has occurred, she continues to experience occasional discomfort and is unhappy about her inability to resume her running just yet. To deal with this she starts with a visit to me and follows with physical therapy, orthopedic visits and finally a chiropractor to correct a problem which would ultimately resolve on its own. While this goes on, she is devastated by her inability to resume running and its effect on her fitness and body image. I try to explain that injuries take time to heal, but she feels something should be done. Medicine should be able to help. "If they can put a man on the moon..."

I don't for a moment diminish the inconvenience and discomfort experienced because of colds, twisted ankles, upset stomachs, backaches, headaches and the like. I have a busy schedule and I understand the problems created when my schedule is altered by illness or injury. These are real problems and cause real suffering. The important distinction is that most of these will get better if left alone or treated with limited efforts to relieve discomfort. More important, because of their transient nature, they do not require massive expense and medical attention to alter their course. Treatment can be expensive and in most cases, does little to speed recovery. Moreover, the treatment can sometimes be worse than the problem for which it was intended.

Few if any simple answers exist. If we have learned anything about scientific advances, it is that each new change creates new problems and risks. Medicines to lower cholesterol can inflame the liver and muscles. Spectacularly successful treatments such as bone marrow transplants for leukemia and lymphoma can lead to new cancers later in life, and impose burdens and added risks not present before these treatments. Coronary bypass surgery can cause strokes and other complications and doesn't always return people to productive and rewarding life. Chiropractic manipulation often provides relief from pain, but it can sometimes damage the spine and nerves and has occasionally caused strokes. Herbal medicines taken by an unwitting public who believe that because its herbal, its safe, have led to many cases of liver and kidney failure, muscle inflammation and seizures. None of these options, as well as the many other alternatives, are perfect. All remedies are associated with risk and the potential for benefit or harm.

The health care industry stands to gain by a health obsessed public. A trillion dollars were spent on health care last year. This money went to hospitals and their employees, doctors, medical supply and equipment manufacturers, pharmaceutical companies, insurance companies and their employees, alternative medicine providers, chronic nursing facilities, advertising and public relations companies, employees of the federal and state regulatory agencies, medical waste handling firms, and many others. Some of this money clearly supports our economy and provides jobs to millions. Much of it pays for necessary health care. However, worry and hype drive up the cost of medicine enormously through unnecessary office visits and tests, operations, medications and hospital stays. Fortunes have been and continue to be made by people and corporate entities at all levels without improving the quality of health care or its accessibility to the general public.

Certainly the medical profession shares a large burden of blame over the last three generations for seeing people as illness waiting to happen. Medical training has taught that patients exist for us to find something wrong which we can diagnose and treat. We have built enormous edifices designed for health care to search out and treat the most elusive diseases. My medical training taught me to be alert for "great cases", usually defined as patients with puzzling and frequently awful diseases which I found by careful sleuthing and often expensive lab tests and investigations. Health care providers as well as the institutions with which they are affiliated reap greater profits as ever more warm bodies come into the system.

A physician I knew saw patients as an income stream that could be tapped into through the use of his laboratory and x-ray facilities. If the x-ray equipment broke down, he could simply perform more laboratory tests. When one part of the process became inactive, the income stream could be maintained by simply increasing the use of another. This concept of the medical office as a cash cow has been usurped by the modern health care industry with medical centers and nationwide medical corporations tapping into this income stream by developing efficient profit centers which capture patient lives like a commodity.

At the same time, we have deluded people into believing that all of this high power and expensive medicine is essential to protect health and survival, thus maintaining the supply of worried patients. We have fostered the belief that in order to be on top of your health, you must have lots of tests and attention from the best doctors, use of the newest technology and access to the biggest names in medicine. We have trained the population to view themselves as patients with potential diseases rather than as people who are occasionally inconvenienced and sometimes disabled by illness.

With all these forces marshaled at focusing attention on health, illness and the desire to prolong youth, it is no wonder that the public is driven to find the cause and cure for every ache and pain. They are led to believe by the entire medical industrial complex they can be the character in the advertisements, the picture of vitality, if they would only make use of these marvelous services. The secret truth is that most of us don't need all this medical care. For the overwhelming majority of people a cold is just a cold, a backache is only a backache and a headache is just a headache. We don't need to rush to the doctor, chiropractor, herbalist or emergency room. With a little insight and patience it is possible to avoid becoming a patient. In the chapters that follow I try to shed light on some of these issues and suggest how not to be trapped by obsessive and unrealistic fears of illness and equally unrealistic expectations of health care providers and technology.

# 3

## "I'M SO FAT"

A middle-aged woman whom I have cared for in my practice for over ten years shows up two and a half years late for her annual physical. She is tastefully dressed in hanging clothes and striped patterns carefully chosen to cover her excess weight. She smiles in a disarming manner, but her obvious flush and rapid speech reveal her to be anxious and obviously uncomfortable as she fidgets about in her seat opposite me. She begins by saying, "You're going to yell at me." She flushes and her eyes swell with moisture. " I couldn't come to see you until I followed your advice and lost some weight. I'm afraid I haven't done a very good job of it. I was just too embarrassed to come in." Clearly, had we not sent her a letter that she was overdue for her mammogram, she still would not have made an appointment.

I try to minimize her fears by reminding her that she is not a fat person but a person who has many health issues, one of which is her weight. Despite my efforts to change the focus of our discussion to other aspects of her health, it is clear that she is still upset. I remind her that she has not had a Pap smear, stool blood exam, blood pressure check, breast exam or mammogram in almost three years, and we need to focus on these issues first. In the examining room she is hesitant to get on the scale. "You're not going to make me do that, are you?" Of course, I don't yell at her as I do not yell at any of my patients, though I do ask her to get on the scale.

Patients' behavior in the examination room is always a source of interest and information. Some are on the scale before they begin to change or the moment they remove their clothing. I can hear the metallic clank of the scale through the examining room door. Others, like this patient, manage to avoid contact with the device which might demonstrate to them and to me their inability to lose weight, as if I would not discover their perceived failure without this tangible confirmation. Several studies confirm that active avoidance of the scale or an unwillingness to comply with a request to be weighed represents a significant sign of problems with body image. The whole business becomes sort of a psychological dance as I explain the need to document weight change to understand any processes going on in her body. At the same time, she presents me with a series of reasons for not documenting the weight, followed by an almost pleading request not to make her get on the scale. I used to argue the issue until I gained enough wisdom to recognize this as classic avoidance behavior. I don't press her, and at her request, I use her own scale weight at home for the record. She is clearly overweight by the standard charts. "You need to get bigger gowns, doctor." She is uncomfortable being seen in a cloth johnnie that barely covers her form, though I use very large gowns expressly for this reason. I find it curious that those whose weight prevents reasonable coverage are unable to acknowledge that the gowns are small because the patient is big.

It is obviously more comfortable to transfer the responsibility for the undersized gown to me, rather than confront the oversized body. We move on with the examination and later return to my office where I try to explain to her that her anxiety and low self-esteem are of greater concern to me than her body weight. I point out that neglecting important aspects of health care because of concerns about her weight is not only misplaced concern, but also dangerous. We then discuss her reasons for failing to achieve her obviously important goal of weight loss. She then admits to me that she does indeed enjoy eating and yet wants to look good. She doesn't want to diet, but she wants to fit into her ideal self-image.

I try to point out to her, as I do with others; the conflict inherent in this common wish, though my success is limited. It is curious how reasonable persons could be satisfied with their actual body in a culture which worships the thin perfectly proportioned cover-girl look or the muscular athletic form devoid of excess fat. While the fitness and diet industry hammers away at our psyche, the food industry drums home its picture of pleasure and gratification. Both are equally skilled in delivering their overt, subliminal, and conflicting messages.

Who could resist the temptations advertisers for restaurants offer us? Dripping fudge sundaes, thick juicy burgers, sweet fried chicken and wonderfully delicious chocolate bars? But, when was the last time you saw an advertiser show an overweight person eating any of these delights? We forget that we can't have both an unrestricted diet and weight loss, though somewhere deep in our psyche we acknowledge this truth. You can't have your cake and eat it too without expecting to put on weight. When you look in the mirror at night, there is that brief moment of reality when you admit how the extra pounds got there. How can you succeed in carrying that awareness over night into morning and sustaining it through the next 24 hours until you once again look into the mirror and say "I was good today" rather than "Why can't I lose weight? Why am I always fat?"

As a doctor, my concern is focused on those people who actually try most of the time to watch what they eat and swear that they don't eat much. Nor do they believe that they eat more than their thin and trim friends. Their standard response when I ask if their diet is going well is, "I don't eat a thing. Honestly!" Now, of course, I know that they do eat well, since I have been with many of my overweight patients at social functions and dinner parties. I have been known in the past to raise my eyebrows as they filled their plates at the buffet or sampled tentatively from the desserts. I have watched them avert their gaze or try to eat out of my line of sight. It has become a source of humor and a source of embarrassment. Over many years, however, I began to notice that, in truth, they were not eating more than the thinner patients or friends or even more than I.

What has became obvious to me is the similarity in populations of people who are overweight. The more of this similarity I saw, the more I realized that this tendency seemed to run in families. Overweight patients often accompany their overweight children or parents to my office or appear at other times for visits of their own. In some cases, I have watched previously trim patients become overweight as the years pass, assuming the body habitus of their parents I had cared for in the past. It is so common in spite of all their efforts to avoid the presumably predetermined outcome, that I can almost predict the change in some families. Occasional obvious exceptions to this pattern often have other characteristics that make them seem different from their heavier relatives. They are taller or shorter, blonder or darker, rounder or narrower in face. But in any event, they are different. If they are not different in appearance, then they are different in behavior in that they are obsessive and almost religious about their attitude towards diet and exercise. They manage to overcome what appears to be a hereditary tendency by modifying their behavior in an extreme fashion.

This difference confirms my impression, now slowly being supported by medical research, that there is something biologically different about people who become fat when caloric supplies are unlimited. I call this the Efficiency Theory of Weight and Energy Balance. In essence, I believe that people who have this tendency to overweight need fewer calories to sustain their normal biological functions than people who are thin. That is to say, they are more efficient in their use of energy. This is very likely based on the efficiency of their mitochondria.

The mitochondria are the structures within all cells in the body which take the calories brought into the body and convert them into high energy bonds which are used as the power source for all the bodies reactions. This includes making and repairing new structures, powering the formation of important chemicals and hormones, facilitating the movement of muscles, transmitting information through the nervous system, and thousands of other activities. An efficient energy generator requires limited amounts of fuel (calories) to perform required activities. On the other hand, the inefficient pumps require lots of calories to keep the generator and the factory going. Fat people, I believe have efficient generators. Thin people have inefficient ones. If people in the efficient category eat as much as those in the inefficient, they will have lots of excess calories to store away as fat. Though the biochemistry involved in this process is complex and only now becoming apparent, the message is simple. In the United States at the end of the twentieth century, except for those unfortunate millions who don't have enough to eat, we are living in a setting of excess available calories. Hence, lots of overweight people.

From a Darwinian perspective, the predilection to efficient energy pumps must have some evolutionary value. I tell my overweight patients that they must have had some ancestors back in the forest, jungle, desert or swamp who had a significant advantage because of their ability to survive long periods on limited amounts of nutrition. This genetic characteristic was transmitted down through generations because of the advantage it bestowed on descendants.

For all we know, it may still confer some survival advantage, though the manipulation of evolutionary pressures by modern science may have changed this. The important point to be made is that this tendency to being overweight is primarily, though not entirely, biologic and not behavioral. I believe strongly, based on more than 20 years of practice and observation, that it is indeed much harder for some to lose weight than others. In other words, it's not your fault.

By attempting to lift a sense of guilt I do not however eliminate the danger of excess weight and its effect on health and survival. In those patients whose excess weight leads to high blood pressure, diabetes, arthritis in the weight bearing joints, increased risk for heart disease and general debility and weakness, there must be a recognition that although the task of achieving weight reduction is difficult, it is not impossible, nor is it unachievable. Like the exceptions to the familial grouping which I described earlier, these people can achieve effective and sustained weight reduction and improved fitness if they make changes in their behavior. This approach runs counter to the natural tendency to consume limited calories. In other words, they must become obsessively fanatic about their diet and exercise. If their thin friends can get by on 45 minutes of exercise 5 times a week and 1200 calories a day, they may need two hours of exercise and 800 carefully balanced calories. This is obviously a major commitment in time and mental energy that some are willing and can afford to make.

A recent patient went through the same series of protestations and discussions outlined above in the first patient until I got to check her blood pressure, at which time I found that for the first time the numbers indicated the development of high blood pressure. It was clear at this point that the issue of weight had become more important. I explained to her that we know from studies on large numbers of patients that up to a third of patients who present with a new finding of high blood pressure can overcome this problem with an increase in aerobic exercise, increased consumption of fruits, vegetables and fish, reduction in dietary fat and salt consumption, and moderate weight reduction. I offered her the option of working on her diet and exercise instead of going on medication. As expected, she chose to try to control this with her own efforts. We were faced with achieving a goal which had eluded her in the past. Because of her previous difficulty, I urged her to participate in a structured program of exercise at her local gym with regular visits to see me to document her progress. An appointment was made with a nutritionist to review her diet and plan a sane approach to food selection. We set modest goals which she found acceptable, and she left determined to overcome the blood pressure on her own. This time, fortunately she was able to normalize her blood pressure while making some major life style changes. Given the pressures of life and the difficulties incorporating all these changes into a daily routine, many cannot achieve a sustained loss of weight. Therefore, they are destined for disappointment in their efforts to avoid medical intervention for the various complications of obesity.

In an effort to get around this limitation, millions have turned to outside help. As expected in our consumer culture, a multibillion dollar diet industry flourishes in response to the seemingly unlimited demand for help with weight control pushed by the continuing cultural emphasis on youth and appearance. Four different approaches are available:

1. Nutritionally complete manufactured diets
2. Diet support groups
3. Spas
4. Medically supervised weight loss programs (inpatient and outpatient)
5. Counseling to deal with issues of body image and self esteem

The manufactured diets are easily available through supermarkets, health food stores or home marketing groups who reach you either through friends or at your work place. These concoctions are purchased either as a powder or as liquids, or come as fully prepared meals. The daily caloric intake is strictly regulated and adequate nutrition is assured if the full portion is consumed at each meal. Some of these are quite artificial in their taste and consistency and others have all the appearances and taste of a normal meal. With some you can simply pop the package right into the microwave. The whole process is quite simple. There's no planning or thought necessary other than to choose the can, powder or freezer package. If followed carefully, nearly anybody can lose weight on these programs.

Why, then, is it so rare that I see any success with this approach to diet? Why do I hear patients so often say, "I tried all that stuff. It worked for a while, but I gained it all back"? Part of this is due to the fact that we're all human and most people can't resist the urge to "cheat" once in a while. Unfortunately, once in a while is more often than we recognize or admit. A low fat cookie or a dish of low fat ice cream or yogurt is just unavoidable, and low fat does not usually mean low calorie. These products usually have lots of calories in the form of carbohydrates or protein. Moreover, after a while the manufactured diet programs become boring. In the real world, people feel the need to eat real food. They need to feel normal.

Diet support groups can be very useful in that they offer guidelines and the strength available from identification with others with a shared problem. They provide the struggling overweight individual with a sense of fellowship and encouragement. The positive feedback delivered with each weekly increment in the battle against the scale is probably one of the most effective devices available to those committed to the process of diet and weight loss. Unlike the manufactured diets, however, the support groups demand more self-discipline and control in planning meals and choosing food. Witnessing the failures of others can be discouraging. On balance, these programs are good and I try to encourage patients to participate if they are able. They often respond to this option in the same manner. "Oh yeah. I tried that. It worked for a while."

Spas have become popular as another method for achieving weight loss, though mostly for the wealthy. In the remote past, they were a place for the upper class to be pampered and massaged. They represented an escape from society and the consequences of self-indulgences. Today they flourish as a place where those concerned about diet and weight control can turn over responsibility for their bodies to the watchful eyes of dietitians, exercise therapists, meditation counselors, aerobic instructors, aestheticians and other similar care-givers. It's a luxury somewhat like sending your Mercedes in for its annual check-up to keep it running smoothly and to maintain the warranty. Their educational message is solid as they emphasize proper diet and moderate exercise as part of the keys to a healthier life.

Often, some of the more health-oriented spas will provide a cardiovascular and fitness profile before and after participation in one of the expensive two to four week programs. These will clearly demonstrate in most cases how compliance with the rigid program at the spa lowers the levels of cholesterol and other blood fats, improves HDL or so-called "good" cholesterol, improves exercise capacity, and provides an overall improved sense of well being. Unfortunately, once most of these patients return to the real world, they resume their old ways. For some this may be immediate, while for others it can take months for the habits to return.

A particular clinic affiliated with one of the most well known universities on the southeast coast of the United States has a large cadre of people with severe weight problems who return on an annual basis. They are placed on an ascetic diet of rice, vitamins and a few other supplements. They drop a few pounds and commune with familiar friends in the same dilemma, then return to their homes all over the country where they resume previous dietary and exercise habits and rapidly regain weight.

One patient with hypertension, diabetes, sleep apnea and degenerative arthritis of his knees travels regularly to the Pritikin clinic in Florida, one of the more aggressive and medically oriented spas. He always returns with spectacular improvement in all of his laboratory parameters, feeling energized and committed to a healthier life style. He also routinely falls off the fitness wagon within a few weeks. By his next visit, he is usually back where he started. When he returns to see me he is filled with shame and embarrassment due to his inability to sustain his progress. As in the case of the nutritionally manufactured diet, people need to live, exercise and eat in the real world. While the coddling and counseling of the spa life has short term benefits, for most people, those who need to change the most, it accomplishes little in the long run except to increase their sense of guilt when they slide back.

The medical profession has risen to the occasion, both out of a desire to help those who suffer from the physical and emotional impact of being overweight and out of a recognition of the monetary rewards available to those who tap into this lucrative market. A generation ago, those who pandered to this demand by seeing patients for weight control and dispensing diet pills were disparaged as "diet doctors", particularly by the medical community. It was believed that the medications they used were potentially dangerous and usually ineffectual in the long run in spite of some short-term benefit. The image of this lowly regarded but much sought after medical doctor doling out pills to suburban house wives has been replaced by an academically and professionally respectable group of nutrition and weight management experts, many of whom give out medications which are potentially dangerous and often ineffectual. These doctors now promote medically supervised weight management programs with all different varieties of liquid supplements, planned meals, vitamin supplements, behavioral management seminars, and now pills. They have mostly given up on the surgical management of obesity with wired jaws, procedures to exclude part of the gastrointestinal tract from functioning with resections and stapling, balloon placements in the stomach and other dramatic but ultimately risky or unsuccessful approaches. Now, most of them will quote highly successful figures representing their achievements in reducing weight under medical management. Some will even project results out for up to two years in order to overcome the well-documented evidence that the true long-term success rate of these programs is on the order of five percent.

The most lucrative diet industry is directed at the general market. Self-help publications line the shelves of bookstores and supermarket check out counters. (I often wonder if they should be placed at the check in counter along with the carriages.) Tabloids and magazines, particularly those directed at women, announce the latest miracle diet to enable you to lose 10, 15 or 20 pounds fast without really trying, often with spectacular before and after pictures. If we would just follow the plan, we will be able to fit into that trimly cut new suit or that slinky new dress just like the ordinary person in the advertisement. Of course, the ordinary person doing ordinary things in the ad is in reality one of those select few models who make it past the ordinary rest of us because of their remarkable good fortune of anatomy and an obsessive commitment to maintaining it.

I see frustration and sadness every day in the eyes of those who view themselves as failures in this battle against weight. Fashion magazines, television shows and the movies present images unattainable to most and can only lead to a loss of self-esteem. Although counseling is available to help combat the inevitable sense of failure in the face of the media image of slimness, few take advantage of this option. Alternatively, while psychiatric counseling and therapy might be considered, success is too often measured in pounds rather than in self-value.

One patient who stands out was a woman who weighed more than 250 pounds on her short frame. She was one of the most joyous and exuberant people I have ever known and her presence in a room was more notable for the spirited intellectual discussions she prompted than for the physical presence of her size. Her radical commentary on local and national politics was always sure to stimulate a vigorous discussion, and she never left without recommending a book, play or movie. She made light humor of her weight and truly enjoyed eating. I looked forward with pleasure to our professional and social encounters and considered her to be a close friend.

Unfortunately, she developed an unforeseen and rapidly progressive cancer. As the disease spread over two years she became wrongly, overwhelmingly guilt-ridden that she had brought this on because of her obesity. With each new symptom of tumor, she bemoaned the fate to which she had sentenced herself. In spite of all my efforts and those of her oncologist to dissuade her from her mistaken belief, in the end, she focused all her despair and anger about her illness on her weight and became ashamed and isolated. She discouraged visitors and sought out ever more punitive treatment programs to try to arrest her cancer, leading to progressive weight loss and wasting. Though she appeared gaunt and starved towards the end, she continued to see herself as a fat person who was being punished for her inability to control her appetite. This was an existential wrong inflicted on this patient by her internalized societal values about weight and body image. When she accepted her weight as her natural condition she was happy and satisfied with herself, but once she focused her anger and despair about her illness on her weight problem, she was lost.

While I was in the process of writing this book, I was asked to see a professor from a local university. She was in her mid-forties and massively overweight. Like many women, her weight problem began with her first pregnancy and rolled right along into and beyond her second pregnancy. In spite of a multitude of attempts at various diet programs, she managed to gain over 100 pounds from her wedding weight. She was so ashamed that she couldn't face a physician for more than 10 years. Her colleague who had requested that I help with her problem presented her to me as a brilliant scholar, a leader in her field.

As she entered my office, I must admit, I was more than a little uncomfortable with the air of suspicion and dread which she seemed to carry. She was consumed with a sense of worthlessness and fear of rejection in spite of an impressive academic reputation. We discussed her work and an upcoming book she was completing, and it was clear this was a source of pride and accomplishment. She relaxed even more when we began talking about our children and our frustrating and often comical experiences dealing with an adolescent daughter. I found myself losing my initial uneasiness in her presence as we established a connection. Once again, as often happens when I meet new patients, I felt as if I were acquiring a new friend. She was able to tell me that her concern was the excessive weight and it's potential effect on her overall health and her ability to function in her work and as a mother.

As she began to tell her story of diets and failures, her mood changed and she wept. It pained me to see such anguish. I took some time to explain my theory about obesity. With strong emphasis on acceptance, I let her know that I did not see her weight problem as a sign of character weakness. There was a distinct change in her mood and facial expression as I launched into my story about ancestral behavior and genetic patterns. When I told her that I sincerely believed that it was not her fault, she seemed relieved and animated to the point that we were able to move on to more significant health issues. When we finished our visit, she left the office uplifted, not because of any special magic or great intellectual skill on my part, but because she felt vindicated and accepted.

The anxiety experienced by my patients, a form of self-flagellation which I have heard hundreds, perhaps thousands of times is instructive. It is emblematic of an attitude towards weight and body shape which affects our self-image and our relationships with others. Somehow, we have come to believe that being fat is a characterologic defect akin to our conception of alcoholism, drug addiction, or gambling. It is seen as a sign of weakness or sinfulness that could be resolved if only the fat person would learn to control his appetite. When they fail, as will be the case in the long run most of the time, the anguish which results is destructive to any sense of personal control. In short, it is an assault on the ego. It is high time for overweight people to stop feeling guilty about their weight. Some of the most wonderful people I have known have been significantly overweight, but did not let it alter their ability to gain happiness from the world. Their weight was an issue for others, not for themselves.

The message to the chronically overweight should be, "It's OK". Although it's true that excess weight is a risk factor for many important diseases and I continue to encourage aggressive weight loss and exercise, if your choice is not to diet, then stop fretting. If your mother or spouse or employer insist on being upset, that's their problem not yours. Get on with your life. Stop worrying about it. Stop reading glamour magazines that are designed to make you feel inadequate and instead deal with the important issues in your life- your children, your job, your society. Learn to be happy with yourself as an individual made up of something more than fat cells. In your case, my job is to take care of you and help you deal with the medical complications which might arise from your weight problem, not to pass judgment on your decision. Be prepared to accept the consequences of that excess weight. If, on the other hand, you want to make a life long commitment to weight reduction, that's great. I will help to the best of my ability using the principles of good medical practice. Remember the process always requires a sustained drive over many years to maintain the changed life style. Without this, the weight will gradually return.

Serious weight reduction is in fact possible with the appropriate level of desire and commitment. There you are, standing in front of the full-length mirror and looking at your sagging waist line, buttock and thighs. Your face is rounder than you remember and you'd like to see some of those muscles you know are hiding underneath the fat. You swear that you've had enough and now things are going to change. At this point you need to consider several issues and make a number of important decisions. First, do you really mean it? You should not underestimate the magnitude of the commitment required. Second, are you willing to forgo the culinary pleasures with which you will be constantly confronted. Third, can you take the heat?

While having a bagel and my decaf coffee in the hospital cafeteria recently, I bumped into Joe, a 64 year old executive who was completing his last week of curative radiation for early prostate cancer. He looked remarkably well, and reported no problems with his course of treatment. He was particularly proud of his weight loss which he had aggressively pursued once he was confronted with the fleeting nature of his existence. The only disappointment he felt was the reaction of his friends who expressed compassion and consolation when encountering him at work. They saw his weight loss as a sign of the cancer and treatment effects, rather than as evidence of his improving health. Another patient, a gay man in the travel business was told to diet because of the new diagnosis of diabetes. Rather than being congratulated for his success, he was more typically gently soothed by friends who saw his weight loss as a sign of AIDS. Don't underestimate the negative impact of people's reactions to your changed appearance.

Assuming the answer to all these questions is "yes" and you're being honest with yourself, you need a plan. Consider where you can cut excess calories. Many patients who want to lose weight will ask me for a diet or a referral to a nutritionist. I ask them to tell me if they know what they're eating that they shouldn't. In almost every case, the answer is an obvious yes. Whether it's desserts, too much bread, portions that are too large, too many chocolate bars, or just too much junk food, most Americans can quickly identify the source of their excess calories. That's 50 % of the battle. The other 50 % involves giving up these treats which have become a habit and a source of gratification. It can be done. I've seen it over and over again—but it's not easy. Weight loss cannot occur without a regular program of aerobic exercise. The key to dieting has to do with burning up more calories than you take in, so daily exercise is critical. You should choose an exercise plan that you can follow. Don't expect to go out and run for an hour a day, shower and change if it will not fit into your schedule. Going to a gym where you can get supervision and support is a terrific idea if you can afford the price and can commit yourself to going on a regular basis. I like to recommend home based exercise, because there is no excuse for not going. All kinds of devices are available inexpensively either new or used that can be operated in the home for twenty or thirty minutes a day with no disruption in your schedule. The key to making this work is commitment to the process.

Set reasonable goals. Many patients will tell me they intend to lose 60 or 70 pounds by a certain date. I tell them to make it twenty pounds and shorten the time period. Anywhere from one half to two pounds a week is reasonable. After you lose the first twenty, the next round is easier. Once a successful routine is established, the problem becomes more one of controlling your behavior so that it doesn't become an obsession. Rather, the goal should become one of life style change so as to maintain the weight loss. Every study looking at long term success and failure of diet programs of all types shows clearly that diets which are not accompanied by modification of behavior will fail in the long term. The common phenomenon of wide swings in weight as people gain and lose from one diet program to another is distinctly unhealthy and only adds to the sense of worthlessness and failure.

I vividly recall one patient, a 34 year old man who was overweight and out of shape with high cholesterol, high blood pressure and very limited exercise ability. When given the choice between medical therapy and changed life style, he stopped smoking, began running and working out at a local gym and is now a trim long distance runner with normal blood pressure and cholesterol. Several times a week he spends hours working out at the gym and running on the street. His diet is as strict as the most carefully supervised nutritional program. He changed his life by determination and desire.

Just like medical treatment, however, even this option has potential side effects. His wife could not adapt to his new life style and their marriage, already slightly strained, was now threatened with disruption. Her calls changed from appeals to encourage him to take better care of himself, to requests for a more balanced pursuit of health at the same time as advice and referrals for counseling. Now he has moderated his exercise program significantly, sees a marriage counselor regularly and has a healthier though perhaps not as physically fit a life as before.

I have seen many patients choose this course, but even more who do not because their motivation and life style could not tolerate the changes needed. Try as they might, they cannot achieve the weight control they so desire. At some point we have to say to them, it's not your fault. I tell my patients that diet and weight control is a large task which can be achieved by some but not by all. Until we find a better way to physically, chemically and mentally control behavior and metabolism, you should worry about the things in life that you can control. Don't waste your money on expensive programs and medical treatments. Don't let the enormous diet and medical industry turn you into a targeted consumer. The solution comes from inside you. If you can fit regular exercise into your schedule and modify your eating habits for a long time, you may be successful. But if these goals are inaccessible due to the press of home and work responsibilities or emotional issues, don't let the concern over weight govern your life. When you look in the mirror, don't see a fat person. See a person who among many other traits also happens to be overweight. Learn to emphasize the valuable aspects of your character and don't allow yourself to be a victim.

# *4*

## RUN FOR YOUR LIFE:
## THE DRIVE TO EXERCISE

At 35, you find yourself working harder and harder to keep up at your job. In order to stay above water you have to keep longer hours, leaving the house earlier and getting home later. You may even be working two jobs just to keep the bills paid and have enough left over for some discretionary entertainment. You get home at night, hopefully in time for dinner with the family, help with homework, pay the bills, perhaps talk to a relative or friend or deal with the latest family or social crisis. It's almost 10 PM and you're ready to drop. Or perhaps you have been at home all day dealing with the needs of three kids, shuttling to school, after school activities, sports events, conferences with teachers, coping with special educational or health needs of your children, running errands to keep the house from falling down, and handling the personal needs of your spouse. Maybe you're older, say 45, and your parents are ill or there is some crisis at work and your job is threatened and you need to consider the progressively limiting options available to you. You sit up at night working on resumes, calling around and trying to network.

At the end of the day, it is hard to think about your physician's advice to get up and work out for 20-30 minutes three or four times a week. You know you want to but you just can't get the physical or mental motivation in gear. You look at the treadmill or exercycle or Nordic trak that you bought with the best of intentions, and you wither, knowing the enticement of a good night's sleep is beckoning. Even worse, you know that tomorrow morning you're going to run into that co-worker or friend who is at the peak of fitness, slim and trim in a Spandex outfit or Italian suit. Television shows and media advertising present you with an array of well conditioned, perfectly muscled bodies They suggest that to live life to the fullest you must be able to wind surf, slam dunk, run the 100, play a hard game of tennis like a professional, or nail a soccer goal with a deft header from the corner. Moreover, to achieve this level of skill and fitness you must purchase their special brand of vitamin, food supplement, clothing, athletic shoes, exercise machinery or thirst quenching liquid.

I do not suggest for a moment that the goal of peak physical fitness can't be achieved. We all know individuals who have followed the current exercise trend to its logical extreme and are now regular participants in marathons, triathalons and long distance bicycle events. I have many patients who are committed to their regular exercise program. Fred, a tax attorney whom I have followed for more than fifteen years, has become a tri-athlete. I often pass him on my drive into the hospital at 5:30 am as he starts his morning five mile run. Another patient who had been quite sedentary and deconditioned, took up cycling and has competed in many annual events covering distances I generally don't drive in an average week. In the course of doing so he has suffered temporarily disabling tendon and ligament injuries, but has persevered. Roughly sixty thousand runners between the Boston and New York marathons are an impressive group indeed. Many thousands more in various events all over the country demonstrate to themselves and others the level of training they have achieved. They find an internal drive and gratification which is worthy of great respect and admiration.

Sadly, most of us barely have time before work each day to walk to our cars or public transportation. We are so cramped by schedules and fatigue that the thought of adding another few hours a week to our responsibilities seems impossible to bear. The spirit is willing but the body is weak. A perfect example is Sandra, a 32 year old nurse who usually comes in to see me with her two small children in tow. The oldest, David, an energetic and talkative three year old, tends to wander about the exam room testing every piece of equipment's ability to withstand his torture while the little one smiles and fidgets in her infant seat. Mom explains how she is desperate to get back into shape since her pregnancies as she reaches down in almost a continuous motion to stop David from destroying my office. She explains to me how her time is cramped with caring for the children, maintaining the house and keeping up her 20 hour a week position as a floor nurse. She needs the latter in order to keep up the payments on the new house into which she and her family have just recently expanded. With her husband traveling several days a week in his job for a local high technology firm, there just doesn't seem to be enough time. Since I'm exhausted from spending only a few minutes in the room with Sandra and her children, I can appreciate her dilemma. I point out to her the obvious fact which she painfully acknowledges. In order to achieve her goal of improved fitness and a more attractive figure she will need to exercise regularly. We both cringe at the prospect of trying to fit this into her day. We discuss diet pills, hiring a personal trainer, joining a gym or purchasing equipment for use at home. Each has it's potential advantage and drawbacks. Diet pills represent a short term inadequate solution to her problem. A personal trainer is obviously too expensive for her limited budget. Clearly, there was no time in her schedule for joining a gym. We settled on finding a used nordic trak for her to keep in her home and iscussed the importance of establishing a firm schedule for its' use.

When I ask patients if they have been exercising, it is remarkable how many people respond that they just signed up at a gym or club a few days or a few weeks ago. They always insist that the timing of this in relation to their annual physical is purely coincidental. By acknowledging the ability to schedule some time for exercise, they admit that the task, though daunting, is achievable. Most of us would love to be in better shape because we all know at some level that we would feel better and be healthier if we could just put a little more planned sweat into our schedules. Fitting exercise into a busy day is just plain hard for the average slug who drags through from Monday to Friday, hoping to hang on to their position or their sanity until the weekend, and nearly impossible for those whose responsibilities last seven days a week. Every once in a while, a patient is astute enough to ask "What do you do for exercise, doc?" I can only meekly respond that I struggle as best I can to get on my alpine tracker a few times a week, often without success due to exhaustion from my work commitments.

We all try to do the best we can. That's not a lot to ask. Unfortunately, a lot of people don't even try. In the course of a normal annual evaluation I ask, among other things, how much do you exercise and what kind do you do? Often patients will sheepishly report that they only walk five days a week or go to aerobics three times a week, when they feel they should be doing more. What they don't realize and I go out of my way to point out is that they are doing more than the vast majority of their friends and acquaintances, or most Americans for that matter. Yet, in spite of their regular and faithful efforts to do something positive, these individuals often feel inadequate under the constant assault of the media hyped image of vigorous and aggressive exercise by the masses. The truth is far from this. Recent population studies show us to be a largely overweight and sedentary society. In view of this, any form of regular exercise, even as simple as a daily brisk walk, is a "step in the right direction."

Very few of us have the time and tenacity required to become a true athlete. On the other hand, patients frequently tell me how much better they feel physically and mentally when they are able to maintain a regular program of exercise. Often they will relate that rather than feeling more fatigued as they had expected, they are able to face the work-week with increased self-confidence and endurance. For a substantial part of the population, the great tired majority, the kind of commitment necessary to reach this goal is difficult. I am more accustomed to the comment of a recent patient who was unhappy with her overall conditioning. "I don't understand why I can't lose weight. I should join a gym or walk at the mall or something, but I can't get myself to do it." Some, out of desperation and inability to organize their time and maintain motivation, will hire an individual trainer to force them to get off their bottoms and do a little work.

We typically drive around the parking lot looking for the space nearest to our destination. When was the last time you walked up the two flights of stairs to your appointment rather than take the elevator which is handily placed to discourage such efforts? Even at my hospital, where fitness should be on everyone's mind, there is no sign directing people to the stairway in the lobby. It is difficult to spot even though it is directly across from the bank of elevators. One patient, a particularly spry 72 year old man, comes to mind. He always walks the ten flights of stairs in his apartment building five times a day for as long as he or I can recall. He walks the two miles from his apartment to my office whenever the weather permits. In spite of a bout of surgery for cancer, he remains in remarkable health on no medications. Another older patient, a woman, has been a long distance walker since childhood when she had no choice but to walk, lacking the money for public transportation. At 79, she is truly physically fit and sees me only once a year because I tell her she must, though I remain unsure as to who benefits the most from our encounters.

These people exercise because it makes them feel good and it has become a part of their daily routine. To walk rather than to drive is simply part of the way they approach life. Exercise for them is not a necessity or an activity advised by their physician or the latest media fad. They are not responding to high intensity advertising by footwear companies or equipment manufacturers. They are not trained as fitness experts nor do they follow instructions from a fitness master. It is just what they do. As a result, their health shows the impact. Their attitude towards life reflects the tempo they create by seeing the world at a walker's pace. They seem to gain special benefits from this pedestrian approach to life. Willie, the father of an old friend, a regular morning walker, came down with a life threatening streptococcal infection known in the media as the "flesh eating" bacteria. He required repeated debridements or surgical stripping of the damaged tissues over many months followed by extensive skin grafting. The ordeal would have been enough to finish off the average 75 year old. This patient, however, survived and recovered completely. Both he and I are convinced that it was his conditioning which largely contributed to his remarkable recovery. The motivation that he had for exercise is similar to that of the previous two patients. Exercise is simply a part of their lives, not something for which they needed to schedule or dress. This is not the "no pain, no gain" group.

There is much we can do in our daily lives to add some exercise into our schedule without significantly compromising our responsibilities or spending a lot of money on medical or other professional supervision. First, however, we must answer the question "Why do I want to exercise?" If the goal is to achieve the level of fitness of the media superstars, our heroes, then the commitment to exercise must represent an obsessive conversion to a life style centered around that goal. More typically the complaint from patients resembles that of a recent 48 year old man. "I'm tired of getting sports injuries. As soon as I get up to the level I should, I strain some muscles. I want the fountain of youth." Very few make it beyond these nascent attempts to become athletes. Every spring I am inundated with patients who become inspired by this model and injure themselves physically or emotionally in their efforts. More often, they become discouraged and quit, unable to reach the idealized image they have created. How often, after watching an athletic event do we, like Walter Mitty, see ourselves breezing along at a blistering stride ahead of the pack to cross the finish line with the tape breaking across our sweaty and heaving chest? With unrealistic images like this, failure is inevitable. The key to gratification through exercise is to set realistic goals. Place the tape at a point where, with reasonable effort and commitment, we can cross the finish line with our lives, families, jobs and self-respect intact.

Healthful exercise does not have to be painful. I often look at the determined and pained expression of some would-be athletes as they trudge by and wonder why they feel the need to suffer so much. I wonder if perhaps this is an acting out of their need to punish themselves for their lack of fitness. Unless they are trying for specific reasons to achieve a particularly high level, such as training for a long distance event or maintaining a competitive edge, valuable and necessary results can be achieved without such discomfort. Simple steps in the course of the day can increase caloric consumption and ask our cardiovascular system to perform more than the usual chair to coffee machine to car to chair to meeting routine.

As a nation we spend billions on exercise clubs, fitness trainers, exercise apparel, videotapes, and equipment. Some of this is well spent, since having the correct footwear and choosing the most appropriate form of exercise is critical to success and avoidance of injury. On the other hand, I could fill a warehouse with all the expensive equipment purchased by my patients which is now either gathering dust in the attic, basement or garage, or serving as a clothing hanger in the bedroom. Similarly, I was recently told by a patient who invests in gyms that one of the keys to their financial success is the enormous number of people who plunk down their membership fee but almost never show up.

Some of the more useful programs springing up around the country now are directed towards first evaluating the individual needs of a prospective client and then developing a plan of exercise which will slowly move a motivated person into a healthy and safe routine. Many of these are carefully supervised and well designed. The clubs often serve as a social gathering place and provide an artificial structure where people can participate without sacrificing their social commitments. Some benefit from the regimented group support of this approach. It is important to remember however, that you don't need a gym to exercise.

At his annual physical a real estate salesman bemoaned achieving his 54th birthday. He complained that he was overweight and out of shape. He found himself getting out of breath carrying his bags in from his car or climbing the stairs in his house. When I asked what he was planning to do about this, he suggested joining a gym near his home, though he had talked of this before and never followed through. I asked, why not go for a 20 minute walk after lunch each day, since his office was in a pleasant residential area in a resort community. "Twenty minutes. I know you can spare twenty minutes. It would also give you a chance to think quietly and in private." It costs nothing and does the job. He admitted this was a goal he could strive towards. We'll see if he follows through.

The key to success in exercising is to make physical activity part of our daily lives. There is no mandatory need to experience pain and suffering in order to reach this goal. The muscles may ache a little, but that sort of discomfort has a positive quality which feeds the feeling of confidence and almost smugness when you've begun to make progress. All that is really needed is desire and a plan. I suggest to most of my patients a determination of what works best for them. Outdoor walking, as already mentioned, is always ideal because it provides the opportunity to bring life back into focus. While exercising the heart and lungs, we can appreciate our place in the natural order while avoiding the cost of the corporate exercise operations. All you need is a comfortable pair of shoes, a light covering appropriate for the weather and an appreciation for the world outside. Whenever I am feeling physically or emotionally overwhelmed I go for a long evening walk and focus on the stars. With my pulse beating and a light sweat breaking, I feel energized when I return to the house. Outdoor walking is also good for the community. Imagine how our cities and towns would change if everybody who was able went out to walk after dinner. I have met some of my closest friends while out walking in the neighborhood. Mall walking is a new manifestation of this kind of activity. Although a far cry from reuniting with the natural environment, this represents an effort by people to return to a more organic form of exercise.

For many, however, walking in the neighborhood or the mall is not a reasonable choice. In that case, two options make sense. Joining a gym with a good program of supervision is a safe and effective plan. Most gyms, both for reasons of competitive pressure and safety, have trained exercise therapists working on the premises. They can provide guidance and a gradual program of increasing cardiovascular work. Programs like this can be inexpensive and are often scheduled at times convenient for all segments of the population. There's also a tribal primeval thrill from squeezing into a gym suit and sweating and grunting together in a group. Why else would aerobic, step and dance classes be doing so well?

If group sweating isn't your ticket, once again I encourage the use of home exercise equipment which combines upper and lower body work, particularly various forms of tracking devices and riding machines. These offer a number of advantages over the gym, particularly if you have reservations about baring your appearance to a large group. The devices can be used on your own schedule with your own choice of music or entertainment to keep you distracted, and you can even keep up with the cable news. I prefer an inexpensive tracker which folds up easily when I'm not using it and can be moved from room to room depending on the activities of other members of the household. If you have sufficient room, there is nothing like a full-blown nordic tracking machine. They can be purchased retail or can be found in the local papers and magazines, often at a substantial savings. Once you get the hang of gliding on it without falling off, the workout you are able to achieve can be set at your own limits. If you have arthritis, joint problems, cardiovascular or other chronic diseases, it's probably a good idea to check with your doctor for any specific recommendations. Remember to start slowly. Many exercise related injuries occur because people have not carefully stretched out and warmed up muscles and joints. Loosen up and build your endurance slowly. Don't expect to work off last night's banquet or the cheesecake you had at lunch by wearing yourself out on a machine.

Think about spending the better part of your lunch break going for a brisk walk or taking advantage of a gym nearby. If you work in any building taller than six floors, stair climbing can be inexpensive and you will be surprised whom you will meet doing the same thing. Try leaving a few more minutes in the morning to walk to work or the train or to a more distant subway stop. Certainly, weather can be a problem. . Nobody likes to arrive at the workplace or school rain drenched or sweaty and out of breath. But it doesn't rain every day. After a few months you will be surprised at how little your breath is strained and how much less you sweat. Safety is , of course, an issue. Choosing routes to walk that are very public and known to be reasonably free of danger is a requisite for any outside walking program. Beyond the potential limitations, there is little excuse other than lack of motivation for not getting at least some exercise on a normal weekly schedule. After you develop a routine, it can become quite an enjoyable habit.

Whether you choose to exercise with others, alone, on the street, in your basement, on equipment or on the floor, the motivation needs to come with a clear understanding of your goals and limitations. Don't permit exercise to become an obsession or allow guilt from lack of persistence to become a burden. If it becomes an obsession, it will displace the mental energy needed to deal with the rest of life.

One very fit 64 year old man said to me, "I'll go run three miles, do 200 push-ups and lift weight for ten minutes, and I feel it's not enough. I used to do more." If you allow guilt and failure to overwhelm you, nothing will be gained and the absence of physical fitness will be compounded by a diminished sense of self worth.

At either extreme, the decision to exercise is something you can do for your health on your own without the medical industry's involvement. Exercise should be something you enjoy that gives you both immediate and long-term gratification. You should not have to go into debt financially or emotionally to achieve fitness or feel a need to comply with some social standard for dress and appearance. The rewards will come not from what people think of your appearance but from the change in the way you feel. Whether or not you succeed at this will depend on your desire and commitment and the plan you create to achieve your goals.

# 5

## OH MY ACHING BACK: SORE JOINTS

I must get five to ten phone calls a day from patients with back pain. They usually start early in the morning as people try to get out of bed after overdoing things a bit over the previous several days. Usually, the plaintive cry is "I can't move. I've been on the floor all night." There is some critical meeting that day, children to be tended, an upcoming vacation or a new job. . "I can't afford to be out of commission today." Inherent in these calls is the belief that I will provide some treatment which will drive away the pain and restore the supplicant to full and immediate function. Sadly, modern western medicine is quite inept in dealing with this common problem.

I try to understand the source and the nature of the pain to be sure there is no pressing medical issue. As a traditional western physician, my goal when faced with this complaint is to rule out any potentially dangerous problem which might require immediate intervention and without which the patient would be in jeopardy. The likelihood of problems such as an impending vascular catastrophe, compression of the spinal cord, kidney stones, or metastatic cancer can be sorted out with a series of questions about the caller's medical history, the character, distribution and onset of the pain. If the story is too vague, a brief examination can often settle the issue.

Once the more serious causes of back pain are moved towards the bottom of the list of potential causes for the distress, I try to reassure that recovery will come and the pain will go away. I point out the inevitable course of an acute attack of musculoskeletal back pain and the meager resources available to ameliorate the caller's distress. I explain that bad things get worse. Less serious problems usually get better. I present a series of guidelines to watch for in the event of lack of improvement. These include loss of control of the bowel or bladder, progressive weakness or numbness in a limb, pain which gets worse when lying in bed, or rapidly increasing or spreading pain particularly in the buttocks. In many cases the pain is sufficiently severe to require a prescription for narcotics, muscle relaxants and anti-inflammatory medications. I present my usual discussion about the utility of limited bed rest which should not last more than 48 hours. Often we end our communication with a sense of incomplete resolution. "Don't I need an x-ray, a CAT scan, an MRI? Shouldn't I see an orthopedist or a neurologist?" I explain that these referrals and tests would be premature at this early stage, since all we would do is proceed in exactly the same manner I'm currently recommending. "Let your body heal on its own," I suggest. Our conversation usually ends here. I can usually tell if I will hear from the caller again.

Much of the fears and many of these calls could be avoided if the injured persons would simply take a few moments to consider their dilemmas before reaching for the phone. How did it happen? What did I do to trigger this pain? Was I exercising, shoveling, moving furniture, carrying, bending or pulling. Does it get worse if I try to move? Has it ever happened before and how did it resolve then? Often, in the course of reviewing all this, patients deny any memory of such trauma until we sit down after the examination. They then recall some activity which they never associated with back pain. "Well, I was roller painting the ceiling and hanging wall paper all day." A recent patient called unable to understand why he had back and shoulder pain. Knowing his work as an artist and sculptor, I asked what project he had been working on. "Right now I'm preparing an exhibition of a new sculpture which hangs from the ceiling, cascading to the floor. Oh," he said, "Do you think standing on a ladder drilling into the ceiling for an hour might have brought this on?"

Sometimes the origin of the pain will be something less obvious, like "I did sleep sitting up in the passenger seat of the car driving in from Cincinnati yesterday." Frequently the pain will come on after a seemingly trivial activity, such as bending to tie a shoe or to pick up the newspaper. These actions do not always, in and of themselves cause sudden back spasm. Often they are much like a match in a tinder box, triggering inflammation and pain in muscles that are so deconditioned or stressed, any sudden load will set them off.

One patient, Lenny is a perfect example. A successful real estate executive, he has suffered from recurrent back problems since his college days. In preparation for major stressful events, whether for business or dealing with his ex-wife, he always develops a sudden spasm of pain in his already unstable back after lifting his suitcase, pulling on his pants or just getting out of his car. If we have an opportunity to speak when he calls for his muscle relaxants and pain medication, I usually ask about the nature of the latest crisis. Fortunately, by now, he is aware of the connection between the stress and his attack of pain. We have not yet gone beyond trying to help him manage stress better. Regardless, he no longer needs to rush in to see me with each episode. He also now accepts the truth that the pain will subside.

All studies have consistently shown that the majority of cases of acute back pain will resolve on their own without any medical, surgical or chiropractic treatment. This is true regardless of whether it is from a strained muscle, herniated disc or "pinched nerve." Most if not all of the money and effort put into medications, physical therapy, manipulations, massage, acupuncture and immediate surgery is likely wasted on achieving nothing or a very short term gain at the expense of increased cost and sometimes increased risk. I do not for one moment question the potential value of all these interventions in giving patients a sense that something is being done or in providing immediate, though short-term relief. While a small percentage of sufferers clearly benefit from some form of directed therapy such as surgery, manipulation or other alternatives, most do not. These therapies, though providing immediate relief for some, do not in general change the natural course of healing.

I would love to be able to send all my patients for a soothing therapeutic massage when they have a back or muscle ache because they would likely gain much immediate relief, though it would be short-lived. Since most patients don't want to pay for this out of their own pockets, this absence of sustained benefit presents a problem. Unfortunately, in these days of cost-effectiveness and managed care, I need to be able to demonstrate to the insurance carrier as well as to the patient that I can change the outcome of the illness with any diagnostic or therapeutic intervention I choose to order. Because the relief is brief and doesn't change the course of illness, it's not a legitimate form of curative treatment from the point of view of those who pay the bill. More important, it does not change the time to recovery or the ability to function during the pain. In the same manner, unless the pain meets some of the criteria I mentioned earlier for more serious causation, radiological interventions of all types, consultations and surgery also have no impact on recovery.

"You mean I have to suffer?" That response stings me, since I understand the predicament. Faced with a patient in pain, it is difficult for me as a physician to accept my limited ability to provide relief. This is sort of a good news, bad news story. The good news is that in most cases, the symptom of pain abates with medications, massage, and acupuncture, The bad news is that there is no reliable evidence that this will change the long-term course of the problem. Some pains get better quickly and others can take a long time. The time required for recovery depends on the degree of injury, the condition of the individual prior to the injury, their pain threshold, and probably many other factors that we don't understand. A small tear of muscle or tendons will take less time to heal than a large tear or big injury to the capsule or sleeve which holds a disc in place between the vertebrae of the back. Either way, healing has to occur, and that healing takes time.

Other factors affect recovery. Most notable are age, conditioning and the amount of continued strain put on the injured area. As we age and our joints wear as they are supposed to, changes occur which damage the structures that hold us together. Much as we might object, our bodies were not created to last forever. The Original Designer made a terrific machine, but for many reasons, just as in modern industry, there is a designed obsolescence inherent in our structure. Parts wear out, particularly those which take the most stress. This leads to changes. Just like shock absorbers, brake pads and ball joints wear out on cars, the discs and supporting structures which stabilize and cushion our backs and other joints wear down. This leads to a loss of the cushioning effect and increased instability with the formation of extra bone in reaction to the wear and tear.

The unfortunate term for all these changes is Degenerative Joint Disease, what the lay public calls "arthritis in my back." Often this can present quietly without creating problems. When a stress or excess load is placed on these joints, whether it is the neck, back, knees, or other important load bearing structures, they are more susceptible to causing trouble, particularly if the joints are not supple and warmed up by conditioning exercises. This is why older, deconditioned and sedentary people or those who have developed degenerative changes earlier in life due to repeated injury, tend to suffer longer with pain. In my early days in practice I found that the elderly tended to live with this discomfort, describing it as "my lumbago" or "my aching back." Now we send these people to neurosurgeons, pain clinics, chiropractors, acupuncturists and physical therapists. We give them pills, stick them with needles, inject cortisone, twist and manipulate them. A few are helped. A few are injured in the process. Most eventually learn to live with the discomfort or to work around the problem.

Thelma is an 83 year old widow who in her earlier days came to see me always dressed colorfully and dramatically made up with bright lip stick and glowing cheeks. She moved with energy and grace. Her greatest pleasure in life was getting out on the dance floor. She would regale me with stories of dancing at the Totem Pole Ballroom and many other clubs in the greater Boston area. She was ageless and appeared as if she would be forever young. As time passed, sadly, her ability to enjoy this activity became limited by progressive degenerative changes in her lower back and hips. Life for her was unbearable. "If I can't dance, then what is the point of living?" I wanted desperately to restore her joyful view of the world. In response to her need for relief we went through all the treatment options described earlier in this chapter. She became despondent and withdrawn. As is often the case, she developed side effects and unpleasant reactions to nearly everything we tried except simple tylenol. Finally, after almost five years, she accepted the truth that her dancing days were over. " I guess if you want to dance, you have to pay the piper," she finally acknowledged. Now much of her vibrancy has returned, tempered by a lot of acceptance and resignation.

We no longer discuss the urgent need to fix and restore youth. She accepts her body as it is, wishes she were young again, but has moved on.

To illustrate the effects of injury and force on musculoskeletal tissues, I often use the analogy of Silly Putty to illustrate to my patients the damage that occurs to body tissues suddenly put under excessive strain. This simple commercial toy can be stretched and pulled into long strands and shapes of all imaginable designs. The more it is worked and kneaded, the more supple it becomes. On the other hand, if it is cold or it is pulled suddenly, it breaks or tears.

Body tissues are very much the same. If they are warmed up or allowed to slowly stretch out, they can perform amazing feats. Stretching to lift the laundry, running two miles, pushing a shovel, reaching for a tennis shot or lifting a mattress to make a bed are simple tasks which should not lead to pain or injury. If the body is asked to suddenly accept a force for which it is unprepared, however, the tissues will give. This is why tension and stress leading to muscle tightening will often lead to injury like the sudden pull on a tensed silly putty ball. The technical diagnosis for the resulting injury is a strain, a tear, a sprain or some similar injury. Once this occurs, there is a natural and healthy response by the body which we call inflammation. The injured tissues respond with the classic four signs which medical scientists define as the inflammatory response- pain, heat, redness and swelling. These are seen by the suffering party as a sign of something gone wrong, when in truth, they are a sign of something gone right as intended. Special cells rush to the damaged area and release a myriad of chemicals and hormones which allow this marvelous system to repair itself. The process is the result of millions of years of evolution and is spectacular to watch at the biochemical, cellular and microscopic level. The initial phase of inflammation takes roughly 10 to 14 days. This is why it takes that long before you begin to feel that the pain is truly fading. Cleanup and formation of new strong tissue to repair the injury can take from six weeks to many months, depending on the type of injury and the degree of healing required.

Patients will often say, "It shouldn't take this long. It's been two weeks already. Could it be something more serious? Once again, they will ask "Do I need to see a specialist or have some xrays or a scan or something?" As long as there is steady improvement and you're doing nothing to prevent healing, it will often take this long or longer if the injury was bad enough. The recovery you experience from the pain you feel after bending over in the garden for a few hours is generally milder and faster than the recovery process from the sudden tearing pain you felt when you were carrying the sofa up the stairs with your cousin who wasn't really holding up her end very well. One represents some mild muscle strain while the other may signify enormous tissue damage and swelling.

It will still be painful when you wake up the next morning or when you get on the plane for your business or pleasure trip. It will still cause you pain to sit in the car for hours, to sit at your desk, or to bend to pick up from below your waist. Sure, a molded plastic back brace will enable you to stand and give that two hour lecture you've been planning for months. But it will not change the fact that time will be needed before you can eventually consider yourself back to normal. Unfortunately "eventually" is a hard concept to accept when you're lying in bed in pain or feel discomfort trying to perform simple daily tasks such as using the toilet, driving the car or tying your shoes. Each hour that passes in this state becomes a source of emotional pressure as well as physical pain. The sense of vulnerability and lack of control brought home by such a seemingly trivial injury can threaten our sense of who we are. This problem is compounded by our cultural impatience with pain and disability. Often, our lives don't allow us the 48 to 72 hours of down time needed to begin the normal spontaneous healing process. When I suggest this brief respite as a method of treatment, the usual response indicates the need for child care, the need to work, the need to meet social obligations. In our fragmented society, many have no nearby relatives or generous neighbors to help.

A common story I hear is that of a young mother who threw her back out bending to pick up toys with a 30 pound child on her hip. That sudden wrenching pain which at first subsides, slowly sneaks back up as the day progresses. The night is spent twisting in bed in discomfort. She forces herself to agonize through the next morning's chores of feeding, diapering, dressing, and cleaning. Finally, desperate with pain, she struggles to the phone and dials the doctor's office. In the background I can clearly hear crying children, a television show, and a distinct tone of anguish in the young mother's voice. I suggest that a brief period of strict bed rest, strong pain medication and mild sedation will likely give her enough relief to return to a limited exercise load for the next 2 weeks. As the words leave my mouth, I realize what a ridiculous suggestion I'm making. Her responsibilities will not take a rest nor will her children's plaintive cries cease for her needs. So I suggest calling a neighbor, a relative, a friend. I am as uncomfortable with my limited ability to provide relief as is my patient with the inadequacy of my response.

Another typical case is the weekend athlete who strains pumping a little more iron than his or her back was prepared to accept. There is no doubt that the pain is real and severe. But there is also little doubt about the folly of trying to play 18 holes of golf the next day or run a few miles "through the pain". People seem to want to test their injury to see if it's better or to see how far they can push without going over the edge. With Monday and work responsibilities looming, a quick fix is wanted. Even worse, vacation may only be days away and the wounded athlete wants to be able to show off the results of exercise and fitness on the golf course, the beach or on the tennis courts.

Mrs. R, a bright and jovial 67 year old woman called me recently with the following story: "I'm sorry to bother you, but my daughter made me call. I bent over yesterday to pick up my grandson and felt something tear in my back. It's worse than the pain I had, you probably don't remember, three years ago. That went away. So I put him down, finished with the few things I needed to do, and called my daughter-in-law to come get little Alex. Since then, I've been lying in bed. I put ice on yesterday, then heat starting today and I started those anti-inflammatory pills you asked me to take before. The pain doesn't seem to go anywhere but my lower back and everything else seems to be working OK. I'm feeling a little better today. I guess I should stay in bed for another day or so, then try to get up, the way you told me last time. If it doesn't get better in a week or so, I'll give you a call. Does that all sound right?"

It certainly sounded right to me. Her daughter, on the other hand, was unhappy with what she saw as the delayed recovery of her mother and day care provider and insisted on a neurological evaluation. This of course included a magnetic resonance image of the lower spine, blood tests for diabetes and bone marrow disorders and a course of physical therapy. Six weeks later she visited me for another issue and wanted me to know that she eventually recovered just as she expected and in spite of all the additional testing and medical office visits.

Most people seem to believe the TV ads which promise fast, fast, fast relief speeding to the pain centers. They show the ailing patient now supple and agile, stretching and sewing, swinging a golf club or bending with a smile to pick up children. Of course this isn't the real world. But the image of quick relief is etched somewhere in our memory banks. The painful truth is, however, that healing takes time, whether it involves an inflamed muscle group, joint or tendon, a herniated disc, a strained ligament or a swollen nerve. The normal intense inflammatory reaction will recede in a few days and then heal slowly over six weeks. As long as the problem is clearly getting progressively better, there is no immediate reason for alarm. When the pain comes for no reason or if it does not start to go away within several days, clearly further medical attention is warranted. In the absence of these complicating parts of the story, the watchword is patience. This too shall pass. It is no wonder that when reassurance is the best I can offer, patients choose so-called alternative forms of treatment. They want something that will promise quick results.

In response to this desire for instant relief, purveyors of cures have proliferated. Chiropractors, acupuncturists, massage therapists, medical back pain clinics, orthopedic and neurosurgical specialty centers all have waxed rich on the pressure created by this demand for relief of back pain. Many of these practitioners are highly ethical and skilled in their fields. Their fame has grown because on occasion, they provide sufferers with dramatic relief. Yet most of them will tell you that in spite of the tilted pelvis, shorter leg on one side, herniated disc, tight muscles or disturbed pain meridians, your attack of acute back pain will absolutely go away on its own if you will simply be patient.

For many of us, there is much we can do to prevent these attacks of pain. Anything that puts excessive poorly directed strain on the back on a continuous basis will tend to increase the risk of back pain. A large overhanging belly, whether from pregnancy or dietary indiscretion, will pull the back muscles in the wrong direction and increase the risk of acute back pain. The former problem will resolve on its own, while the latter will require some effort as discussed in an earlier chapter. Sleeping on your stomach will tend to increase unhealthy forces on the lower back. Deciding on Sunday night when nobody can help that it is finally time to move the old freezer out of the basement by yourself or with your particularly unhelpful cousin is definitely bad for your back. Sitting for hours over a computer keyboard in poor position will also lead to problems in this area. A caller several years ago insisted that there was nothing he had done which could possibly have triggered his severe Monday morning spasm. Fortunately, I recalled an earlier conversation about our mutual sailing interests and his efforts to keep his costs down by doing most of his own work. Since it was the first week in April, I asked if he had started preparing the boat for the upcoming season. He launched into a description of how he was going to beat the boatyard by painting it himself. "So how many hours did you spend bending back as you sanded the bottom?" I asked. The answer was obvious and he knew immediately where I was going with this line of questioning.

One of the most formative events in my career as a physician occurred during a quiet moment in the doctor's lounge at the New England Baptist Hospital, a world renowned orthopedic institution. I was only in practice a year and found myself in the presence of the aging Dr. Ted Potter, one of the giants in reconstructive joint surgery. He, along with others in Boston, pioneered the replacement of injured and worn out knee joints with new metal structures. We were alone and it was late in the evening. The lounge was quiet with low lighting, an excellent setting for introspection and reflection. I could see he was dismayed, nearly in tears. I asked him why he appeared so unhappy. After a sigh and a long pause, he related the story of a close friend and tennis partner who had been slowed by progressive degenerative changes in his knee. Given Dr. Potter's expertise, he offered to restore his good friend's mobility with a new joint. The surgery went so well that his friend soon returned to a vigorous and active life, only to be struck down by a massive heart attack while attempting to play tennis again. Now he lay in the intensive care unit near death. Dr. Potter felt he had been instrumental in his friend's catastrophe by enabling him to resume activity at a point in his life when he perhaps should have been slowing down. I tried to point out that the cardiac event would likely have occurred regardless of his intervention, but he remained set in his assessment of the events. Because I respected his age, experience and wisdom, I will never forget his words before I was paged to a call. "The Lord slows us down for good reason. Sometimes it's best to leave things in His hands."

It seems to me that as a culture, we are either unable or unwilling to accept that the body is not a mechanical machine with parts that can be quickly repaired and replaced like broken shock absorbers or a flat tire. Though I certainly encourage patients to seek care for unexplained and prolonged discomfort, life demands a certain perspective. In short, anything which places unusual or prolonged stresses on the muscles, discs, vertebrae and ligaments will increase your risk of getting into trouble with your back and joints. None of us is immune to this and all of us will at some time in our lives experience an episode of self-induced back pain. We do not, however, need to run for medical attention immediately. Some of the pain will go away with rest and time. If it doesn't, have it checked out by your doctor. While some problems can be fixed or may be due to more serious causes, much of the pain is due to natural wear and tear. Don't assume the worst. Don't rush to the doctor. Try to be patient and maintain some perspective.

# 6

# I'M SO TIRED: FATIGUE

Joe Banks, a young man of about 35, was exhausted. He had difficulty arising in the morning. Five days a week he dragged himself into his boring job at his unpleasant and demeaning work place where he found no reward and no growth. During the weekend he waited to return to the monotonous routine. His eyes felt fuzzy and he had difficulty focusing his vision. He seemed to suffer from a sore throat and a headache almost daily. Pulling at his shirt collar, he peered into the mirror each day, certain that he was unwell. He thought himself to be pale and sickly. He sought medical advice to confirm his fears that he was suffering from some terrible illness. The doctor, who had his own motives, informed young Joe, that he was suffering from a rare and untreatable condition-a brain cloud.

The remainder of the story makes up one of my most favorite movies, Joe versus the Volcano. This existential satire lets us know with tongue barely in cheek that it is rarely the things we fear most which make us feel unwell. The opening scenes epitomize the somatasizing patient. Joe loses sight of the problems which make his life most unpleasant and instead becomes focused on an accumulation of symptoms which make him feel constantly unwell. Provided with a diagnosis which allows him to attribute all his symptoms, improbable though it may be, he accepts a medical explanation for his state of malaise. Instead of brain cloud, one could easily substitute the diagnosis of chronic fatigue, hypoglycemia, or an old favorite from a generation ago, neuropsychologological aesthenia. Without giving away the plot, I can tell you that once he realizes he has nothing to lose, Joe is finally able to find joy and meaning in life, and the symptoms disappear.

Marilyn is a 65 year old woman who has used me as her doctor for 15 years. Although my recollection of all the details of her initial visit is a little vague, two particular aspects stand out both in my memory and in my notes. Like Joe, she complained of tremendous fatigue as she related to me the sad story of her husband's illness. He had been a vigorous and successful businessman who slipped on the ice and broke his neck (technically fractured his cervical spine), compressing his spinal cord and leaving him quadriplegic. He was cared for on a respirator to breathe for him in a nursing home where Marilyn faithfully visited every day. Though she presented a stoic demeanor, it was clear that the burden of the illness and the need to provide physical, financial and emotional support wore her down.

As the years passed, the husband developed recurrent medical crises with infections, respiratory difficulties, and ultimately wasting and death. At the same time, Marilyn had to continue to work and sustain her family. Each year she would come to see me for her annual exam. She always began by saying, "I'm so tired. I have no energy." I would dutifully write this comment into my notes with quotation marks, then listen to her long list of complaints which generally focused on her lack of energy.

In the earlier years I was able to help her recognize the source of her anguish and fatigue. After a careful medical evaluation she could accept the connection between her stressful life and her fatigue. As we both grew older and she acquired medical problems of her own, her symptoms were more difficult to explain away. She developed Bell's Palsy, a paralysis of one side of the face, from which she mostly recovered. This was followed by a duodenal ulcer, thyroid problems, and, most recently, heart disease with angina and an episode of congestive heart failure. These problems are all now well controlled, and yet at her most recent visit she once again began talking about her severe weakness and fatigue. Anticipating my questions, she followed quickly with the protest, "This time it's not just being depressed. Something is wrong. We need to do more testing." As I reviewed her medical problems I found very little going on in the way of active medical issues. I said, "You do seem a little on edge." This was the key to the door.

"I should be on edge, what with my son." I braced myself for this latest calamity in her long saga. "Now that the tumor has been removed from his brain he can begin his recovery at the rehabilitation hospital." She went on to tell me how he had difficulty walking and some problems with headaches and was found to have a benign brain tumor which had grown large enough to compress brain tissue. He had become quite debilitated by this, but there was good hope of a near complete recovery if his therapy went well. Once again, we worked around to try to understand how life's reverses had put a strain on her ability to cope and caused her to experience symptoms which she called fatigue. She always protested her weakness and inability to manage with all these difficulties. As I had done previously, I responded with my admiration of her ability to continue with an active and productive life in spite of the adversity. Her symptom of fatigue was clearly part of her defense against her Job-like predicament. We discussed this and agreed that nothing was new. She would not need all the testing she originally requested.

This type of fatigue is probably one of the most common reasons for seeking medical attention. While this can be the first complaint for many serious medical illnesses, more often it is not because of disease, but rather the result of other factors. A careful physician should never assume the patient's complaint to be without medical cause, though we all make this mistake on occasion. A detailed history and physical examination by a qualified internist or family practitioner with a few simple blood tests should easily rule out the vast majority of illnesses. A few rare conditions may take a little longer to discover. In general, most of those patients who remain after this process and continue to complain of being tired are just that- tired. They drag themselves out of bed in the morning and force themselves through the day's work. By the evening, their spirit and physical strength is flagging, but they push on until they finally collapse either physically, mentally or both. Their fatigue is very real and debilitating and should not be taken lightly by the individual or any physician involved. Often, they have very little insight into the causes of the fatigue and come to the physician anxious to find an answer.

The physician is in a unique position to objectively evaluate a patient's life situation and attempt to focus attention on the underlying problems. People who assume the role of patient when they enter my office have a remarkable ability to drop their inhibitions and unload the most overwhelming burdens in front of me. I hear stories about alcoholic parents, childhood and spousal physical and sexual abuse, bizarre and unwarranted fears about illness, suppressed anger at a spouse, sibling or coworker, fear of failure, fear of success, financial crises, family crises. It seems as though everybody has some awful load to carry. I often find myself looking on my patient in admiration at his or her ability to cope at all given the difficulties they face. And yet, these same people are often unable to make the connection between these stresses and their symptoms.

Before committing to a series of tests, misguided diagnoses and treatments, either traditional or alternative, we need to think carefully about these non-medical causes of fatigue. If the symptom comes on in an unexplained manner and you honestly can find no proximate cause for your complaints, then you should see your doctor. If, on the other hand, you can figure out the problem, resolve it on your own and make the tiredness go away, then you don't need to see a doctor or allow yourself to be probed and prodded, x-rayed and scanned, massaged and manipulated. A few case histories should help to bring this into focus.

Sally is a well-dressed woman who comes in for an annual checkup complaining of a lack of energy. She asks about chronic fatigue syndrome, hypoglycemia or Epstein-Barr Virus infection. She tells of two small children who need to be fed in the morning and then carted off to school or day care, a stressful day at work, then returning home to tend to the needs of her children and her spouse. That's two full time jobs by my book. Sleep is limited by either restless children or the psychic turmoil of her tremendous responsibilities and pressures. Although her voiced concern is of some terrible illness which she may have witnessed in a friend or on television, she readily acknowledges the load she carries and the likely source of her symptoms. Her eyes briefly swell with emotion, but she quickly regains her business-like composure. Fortunately, her history and examination are normal. I reassure her that I expect the laboratory tests will be the same. Since there are indeed no surprises in the blood tests, we talk about her schedule and the remarkable demands she places on herself. I admit that I have always been in awe of the strength and endurance of the working mother. I have no easy solutions, but she finds it useful to talk about the issues and to know that somebody understands her predicament. She vows to take a little time for herself each week, though I doubt she'll carry this off.

Bill D. has been forced by the financial demands of his growing family to assume a heavy load. He works a day job at the local department store and as a security guard at night in addition to going to classes one night a week to have a chance to keep up with the shrinking job market. He's tired, stressed and irritable. He complains that his bowels don't work properly and he has headaches. He has noted increasing difficulty concentrating, and although he is constantly fatigued, he is unable to enjoy a good night sleep. During a detailed history, he reports drinking four to six cups of coffee each day. All other aspects of his medical history are either unremarkable or do not add information to the story. A careful physical examination is unrevealing except for a mild elevation in his blood pressure.

I reassured Bill that on the basis of this information as well as the few blood tests which we sent off, he appeared to be free of any serious illness. Although I couldn't be 100% certain without much more sophisticated testing, I encouraged him to view his symptoms in the context of his life situation. Since I am as guilty as he of overworking, I related to him that my wife often tells me we are not machines and need to take a break once in a while. We discussed a trial period of a modified schedule and an attempt to cut down on his caffeine. I offered to proceed with further testing if his fatigue did not abate in a fixed period of time.

Sally and Bill are examples of fatigue due to pure and simple overload. They ask more of themselves than a reasonable person would ever consider and more than the body was designed to take. As a result, they suffer the consequences. They came to see me worried about illness, but really knowing why they were tired. They either had a need to find some other explanation for their problem which would enable them to go on with their destructive behavior, or more likely, simply needed to be told to change.

In my experience, one of four things will happen at this juncture.

They could accept my advice and begin to readjust their attitude and schedule and actually start to feel better. This is often the gratifying result of a visit. They may not improve in spite of efforts to change all the factors which we discussed, implying the possibility of a legitimate medical problem. They might be disgruntled at another physician ignoring what they perceive as a serious medical disorder and go shopping for other opinions. What is more common, however, will be a continuation of the same difficulties until some crisis forces a confrontation with the need to make changes.

I try to support patients through this process, but I have come to recognize that these changes must come from within the individual. When I am called by a patient's spouse, parent or child asking me to force the patient to change "before it's too late", I often remind them of the well worn truth that you can draw a horse to water but you can't make it drink. While this old saying may be trite, it is rarely obvious to an anxious relative who believes I hold some mystical power to change behavior. It is up to the individual to want to change in order to feel better. No medication, herb, acupuncture treatment or chiropractor manipulation can make this happen.

A favorite patient of mine, a 91 year old gentleman who has seen me only once each year for the past fifteen, comes in for his usual visit complaining, for the first time, of being tired. I have been forewarned about his condition by a concerned niece. He has found it more difficult to walk the three blocks from his apartment to the center of town and he sleeps later than is his custom. Climbing stairs has become intimidating and his ability to clean his home has diminished to the point that he is unhappy with its appearance. He remains bright and alert, and we briefly discuss the current political scene as we often do, though his attention is clearly not focused on such trivial matters. While there are a number of potential medical problems which need to be assessed in a person of his age, careful medical evaluation reveals none of these.

When we sat down several days later to review his results, I focused on his extremely high level of function for the last 91 years, and that perhaps it was time for him to feel tired. He was not happy with this diagnosis. We discussed the alternatives available to assist him in carrying on his level of function, and as expected in such a proud and independent individual, he was resistant to accepting help from others. I suggested that he allow his family and friends to assist him as they are anxious to help. With the encouragement of his niece, I convinced him over the next several weeks to accept help from the local Visiting Nurse Association. Though we were both saddened by this change, we both saw his symptom of fatigue in the context of the life cycle.

The issue of age and fatigue is difficult and often painful. Many vigorous elderly patients often function at remarkably high levels both physically and intellectually. It is not uncommon for me to tell some of my octogenarians that they are the healthiest fifty year olds in my practice. Their appetite and joy of living far exceeds that of many of the younger patients I see, and I relish our visits together. Unfortunately, as time passes, the body and mind slow and their capacity to continue at this high level will inevitably fail. A fall, an illness such as a severe cold or pneumonia, a change in diet caused by poorly fitting dentures can destabilize the delicate balance between slowly declining function and increasing need. Although we recognize this scientifically, it is still difficult for all of us, particularly the children of the elderly, to accept that at some point, part of being old means being a little more tired. Sometimes a nap during the day is more valuable than a trip to the doctor's office.

Mary is a 32 year old divorcee with three children and no job, who complains of feeling tired. I have seen her over the years with various complaints of headache, abdominal pains, muscle cramps, joint pains, sleeplessness and other non-specific symptoms. She ekes by on the supplemental income she receives from the state welfare department and help from her family as well as a few dollars from an occasional odd job. Her sense of self-worth is absent and she finds little joy in any aspect of her life. She has suffered from depression for many years, and has bounced from psychiatrist to social worker to state assigned case worker with little improvement. Her fatigue is palpable and contagious, and I often find I have difficulty staying focused on her latest complaints at each visit. No medical diagnosis has ever been made, since her problems have always been due to her difficult situation and her poorly developed ability to cope. The greatest danger I fear in caring for her and patients with similar problems is losing sight of the important rule that illness can occur in people who display their emotional problems in the form of bodily complaints, a behavior known as somatasization.

Depression is at worst a debilitating and sometimes fatal illness which can masquerade as a multitude of problems, fatigue being one of the more common. Separating these out can be a tedious and demanding process fraught with the risk of misdiagnosis and improper treatment. Often these patients will jump from one physician to another, unwilling or ashamed to accept the correct diagnosis, or dissatisfied with their doctor's inability to deal with the complexity of the problem.

I recall one gentleman, a business executive who was being phased out of his very powerful position because of age and a change in the management of his company. His complaints included cough, shortness of breath, constipation and an overwhelming fatigue. Although he had very mild asthma, it was quite clear to me that he was suffering from fatigue due to his sense of uselessness and loss of power. He was understandably depressed. I tried to reassure him and recommended counseling and perhaps a brief trial of antidepressants, but he insisted that there was an organic basis to his problems. Reluctantly, I launched into a series of medical tests which all proved quite unremarkable. Still dissatisfied with my diagnosis and not a little angry with me, he subsequently visited specialists at medical centers all over the city, undergoing more tests and receiving many different medications. I often heard from his wife who was still a patient. She called frequently with reports of worsening of his symptoms.

To my surprise, he reappeared in my office a year later, still not feeling well, and taking a long list of medications to boot. Under duress, though perhaps more willingly than he would admit, he agreed to visit with a psychiatric social worker. Under her guidance he has come to understand the nature of his depression and, with the help of some medication, he is now dramatically improved and no longer complaining of fatigue. He had believed, with encouragement from a multitude of high priced and renowned specialists that his medical problems and complaints were well founded and in need of treatment. Thousands of dollars and many hours and days were spent chasing his evanescent symptoms. And yet, after a year, we were back where we started, treating his depression and lifting his fatigue.

Michael is a 20 year old college student who was sent in by his parents, concerned about his apparent sleeplessness and his complaints of feeling tired all the time. Their first concern, quite appropriately, was that he had infectious mononucleosis, followed by concerns over all the medical misfortune which can befall a young adult approaching his prime years. The typical worries of a parent in this setting are illness first, followed by drugs. Since he was basically in excellent health, his visit took little time and we were able to spend a while discussing his schedule at college. It came as no surprise to me that he was busy burning the candle at both ends, studying until eleven at night, then going out to party with friends. He often "pulled all nighters" to cram for exams, and then required several days to recover.

As is true at many colleges, alcohol had become a major part of his night life. It was difficult for me to appear too judgmental on this issue, having wasted the first semester of college in a similar manner. I suggested, however, that the student's focus must return at some point and I turned to my standard auto parts lecture. I pointed out that, unlike most objects in our world which are disposable, repairable or replaceable, our bodies come with a limited warranty and very few and costly replacement parts. This is the only one you get and you can't send it back or ask your credit card company to cancel the purchase. So if you're at college and you're wearing yourself down, think about the long-term implications of crippling your only means of transportation into the Big Race before you even get started. I am always startled by how simple and effective this analogy can be, especially with the young. Like children, we need to be told to change our behavior.

Because medical science does not have all the answers and doctors, myself included, do make mistakes, patients often raise questions about some undiagnosable syndrome currently in vogue. During the 1960's and early 1970's it was hypoglycemia which was bandied about as the cause for fatigue in large numbers of people. During the next decade, Chronic Epstein-Barr Virus infection was the most popular diagnosis for people presenting with fatigue. Except in a few very select cases, neither of these has found the degree of scientific support to be accepted as legitimate diagnoses by most of the medical community. The latest manifestation of this phenomenon of fatigue looking for a diagnosis is Chronic Fatigue Syndrome, a disease without a known cause for which there is no known test, and which responds quite nicely in many cases to antidepressant therapy. Its existence is ostensibly supported by the rare patient who has clear-cut evidence of a chronic low grade viral infection. Many of the leading investigators in this field spend much of their time trying to find a test to identify patients with this problem. In general, their results have been disappointing.

A recent tragic case in Massachusetts of a woman who committed suicide to escape from the presumed refractory effects of her CFS illustrates the problem of labeling patients with a disease which can neither be proven nor disproven, cured nor mitigated. According to media reports, her autopsy showed no evidence of any disease process and all her blood tests were normal. Still the prophets of this diagnosis, prominent professors from major teaching hospitals, pronounced her diagnosis to be sound. Like the tailors for the emperor's new clothes, they insisted on the clarity of the diagnosis and how well it suited her. For those of us treating patients like this who suffer terribly from severe and often debilitating difficulties, the diagnosis of Chronic Fatigue Syndrome presents new frustrations in getting patients to address the causes of their symptoms.

All of these examples illustrate a few of the common presentations of fatigue. They could just as easily have led to more serious diagnoses if the examination or tests yielded different results. Fatigue that is unexplained, even in a person who is depressed, whether it be a tired college student, an elderly retired person or an overworked head of household, must be recognized and resolved until both the patient and physician are satisfied with the outcome. Unfortunately for some patients, the symptom of fatigue becomes a chronic complaint. This is usually because of the unwillingness of the patient to accept an alternative non-medical explanation or because of the physician's fear of missing a diagnosis.

Contrary to popular belief, most valid studies have demonstrated a diagnosis in almost all cases of fatigue from among the known medical, behavioral, social and psychological disorders. Despite this fact, people suffering are anxious to grasp at any straw thrown their way which does not conflict with their concept of their condition. Many patients have spent the better part of their lives, in spite of the best medical evaluations and advice, pursuing some unexplained cause for their fatigue. They are convinced that they are the victims of some previously unrecognized syndrome or one of the nebulous non-specific disorders touted by many sufferers. They are encouraged in their search by media stories of rare diseases which are found only after the dogged efforts of the victims. In addition, there are many physicians and para-medical personnel and therapists of various stripes who have made a career and found financial success by pandering to the needs of this group.

If you're feeling fatigued, evaluate your situation first. Are you overworked, over-stressed, taking too many stimulants like caffeine or tobacco, physically abusing your body, depressed or just worried? If you still can't figure out a cause, see your doctor. Once you're confident that a thorough examination and evaluation have been performed, work past the fatigue. In the unlikely situation the symptom doesn't improve over several months, go back to your doctor. Be certain your complaints are listened to carefully and taken seriously. If a further evaluation is unrevealing, don't allow fatigue to be the controlling force in your life. Get to the bottom of the cause and deal with it.

Although a small number of those suffering from fatigue will have something unusual, doctors and patients alike often lose sight of the important rule of logic that rare things happen rarely. Most people are healthy.

# 7

## IT'S NOT THE FLU: COLDS AND VIRUSES

Every day during the cold season it seems I receive endless phone calls which all start the same way. "I have the flu." This can mean anything from a little bit of a runny nose to a full-fledged episode of pneumonia. When asked to elaborate, patients will often pause as if I'm asking a silly question and then respond with a nonspecific series of disconnected phrases to indicate that something is wrong in their body above the waist. It goes something like this: "My ears are... and my throat is arrgh! The congestion. And my body...I'm sure it's the flu or something." This is often followed by a few representative coughs, primarily to demonstrate the nature and severity of their symptoms and also triggered by the constant movement of air over their irritated airway during the brief description. Since patients often mean many different problems when they call their symptoms the flu, I ask for a little more information so I can determine whether this is indeed a simple cold or something more serious. The standard questions include: Are you short of breath? Do you have a fever? How high? With chills? Are you raising sputum and if so, what color? Is there any blood? Do you have pain anywhere? Do you have any major medical problems or take medication on a chronic basis? When the answer to all these questions are negative, as expected, my level of concern drops rapidly.

I don't mean to minimize the importance of a common cold, or to use the more technical phrase, the common upper respiratory virus. Whether it interferes with work or social responsibilities or just makes you feel bad, colds can be a downright nuisance. Rarely, it can even lead to a more serious complication. Most typically the patient will describe a stuffy head, blocked ears, a scratchy throat, mild fever and a slight cough. My initial impulse has always been to say "It sounds like you have a cold. This isn't a serious problem. Why are you calling me for something that will just go away and isn't going to hurt you?" But my training and compassion usually control my cynical side and I appreciate that the call is from somebody in distress who doesn't understand the facts about colds, in spite of having had dozens in the course of his life. This is largely because we, the medical establishment, have for generations, fostered a sense of dependency in the public with regard to illness. Physicians have been happy to keep their offices busy caring for these patients. Pharmaceutical companies, in league with the advertising media have waxed rich selling all sorts of useless treatments. Most of this is unnecessary and occasionally downright harmful. If the public is to learn to deal with the common cold in a rational fashion, they need to know the facts.

For most of the year, the symptoms which prompt anxious calls from patients are not due to the flu and should not cause the kind of alarm they seem to engender. It is helpful to understand that the flu is a distinct illness characterized by high fever, severe headache and generalized body aches, cough, mild to moderate head congestion and frequent chest burning and discomfort. The flu lasts anywhere from a few days in mild cases to as much as several weeks, and then it goes away. Rarely, complications do develop in healthy people, such as pneumonia, pleurisy and some neurologic complications, but there is little we can do to predict who will suffer these difficulties or how to prevent them. It comes only in the midwinter and sweeps around the world in one massive pandemic. When this occurs there is a dramatic increase in the number of hospitalizations and deaths in the community in non-immunized persons who are over 65 years of age, those suffering from chronic serious medical disorders or who are taking medications that put them at increased risk. We know we can significantly protect this high-risk group by boosting their immunity with flu vaccine each fall. The vaccine is developed from fragments of viruses that are expected to be the most likely candidates for the upcoming winter season. We worry about the flu because many people in these groups can and will die from it if we do not immunize. The flu is a potentially serious illness for them, but for the rest of us, we just feel awful but recover usually without any problems. Aside from the well-publicized episode of neurologic problems following the use of the swine flu vaccine in 1968, flu vaccine is safe and effective. It does not cause the flu, nor does it prevent other viral infections.

Often patients will refuse the flu vaccine because they say it gave them the flu or because 20 years ago they got a viral respiratory illness during the week after receiving the vaccine. Since the vaccine consists of fragments of virus and no living viral particles, it would be hard to imagine how this could occur. Infections don't develop from non-functioning lifeless pieces of cells. Pasteur demonstrated long ago that infection was transmitted by living organisms, not dust or magic. I like to point out to my patients that whether they receive the vaccine from me, community health clinics or the local pharmacy, these locations all tend to be areas where large numbers of people who are sick tend to congregate. If they get sick after the flu vaccination, it is more than likely due to the person who was sitting next to them or with whom they shook hands or gave a peck on the cheek hello when going for the shot. You don't get the flu from flu vaccine.

The other more common viral respiratory infections which are the source of so much concern in the public lead to enormous expense and waste. They are also the source of huge profits for the purveyors and prescribers of medicines, vitamins and herbal remedies. If there were any question as to the importance we place on dealing with this problem in our culture, one need only to look at the cold remedy aisle in the pharmacy or supermarket or the cold prevention section of your local health food store. Preparations of all types are lined up in multicolored packages designed to catch the consumer's eye. Their advertisements on television, radio and in the printed media promise speedy relief, and claim this will return the now symptom-free patient to productive activity in no time. What person suffering from a drippy nose, annoying cough, sinus pressure and just feeling lousy would not rush to take such a wonderful nostrum? Who could resist the temptation to achieve such prompt improvement? Why not take some herb or concoction which promises to improve your immunity and prevent infection?

With promises of instant relief, it should come as no surprise to me when a typical patient call comes in. "I'm so sick. I have the flu. My nose is running. My head is stuffy and my throat is scratchy."

I ask, "How long has this been going on?"

The reply causes me to pause. "Since I woke up two hours ago."

I follow with the standard series of questions already outlined, usually with a negative response.

After a moment of composure, I respond "It sounds like you have a good old-fashioned cold. If you feel you need relief from your symptoms, try some over the counter cold remedies and drink plenty of fluid. It will probably last several days and don't be surprised if the symptoms linger for ten to fourteen days."

"Don't you think you should see me or shouldn't I have an antibiotic or something?"

At this point, I usually explain that in an otherwise healthy person without specific symptoms suggesting a more serious illness such as shortness of breath, an unremitting headache, severe shaking chills and sweats, ear pain or other symptoms suggesting a more wide spread illness, it is likely that this is indeed simply a cold. The presumption is usually supported by the presence of such symptoms in large numbers of people in the community. If co-workers are coughing and sneezing and you start coughing and sneezing, the odds are that you all have the same thing. Many patients will respond with "Oh yeah. Everybody at work has the same thing." Unless there is something particularly unusual about your symptoms, it is safe to assume that you have a cold caused by one of many different possible viruses. There is no need to rush to a doctor's office, spend excessively on medications or put yourself to bed for prolonged periods.

People gobble down all varieties of vitamins, herbal remedies and over the counter cold preparations on the belief that they are applying a cure for the infection. Sadly, there is no definitive evidence for any of this. Some recent studies, for example, demonstrated that the symptoms of sore throat and stuffiness responded nicely to the use of zinc lozenges every two hours. This is likely due to an effect of zinc on the bodies immune clearance mechanisms. Unfortunately, the achiness, fever and general lassitude did not last any less long and there was a significant incidence of nausea and a foul taste in the mouth. Antibiotics often cause more trouble than they are worth. While they can be life saving when bacterial infections threaten, they can lead to all kinds of mischief which is unacceptable if there is no potential benefit from the treatment. In viral infections, there is no such potential benefit. In spite of this, modern medicine has conditioned people to believe that a visit to the doctor isn't worthwhile if no prescription is written, or, perish the thought, the treatment is to buy an over the counter medication that could have been started without an expensive and time consuming medical visit.

Antibiotics don't treat colds since colds are caused by viruses and antibiotics don't affect viruses. If you have been or become allergic to the antibiotic chosen you can develop an awful rash or more serious consequences such as liver injury, blood problems or colitis to name a few of the more common complications. Women will often develop vaginal yeast infections from antibiotics which has to be a plain old unnecessary and downright nuisance. Unless the suspicion of a bacterial infection is strong, antibiotics have no place in the treatment of the common cold.

The presence of a fever for 24 to 36 hours in an adult is not necessarily a reason for concern if it occurs in conjunction with these symptoms. Fever is part of the body's response to infection and does not constitute a threat to health except in small children. Some degree of fever is probably necessary to kill off the infection. Many of those familiar symptoms of achiness, fatigue, headache and general lassitude are the effect of the chemicals that the body produces in its effort to limit the infection and destroy the invading virus. I find it helpful to think of the body as a battleground where a war is carried on between the invading virus and your own immune system. The virus attacks cells and tissues in the body which respond with salvos of virus fighting proteins. The two sides duke it out with powerful ammunition and can wreak havoc on the battlefield, occasionally leaving lasting scars. Fortunately for us all, the immune system almost always wins and we recover.

At the onset of typical cold symptoms, many people will take to their beds on the assumption that this will speed their recovery. I often hear the complaint, "I don't understand why I'm not better yet. I've been in bed for five days." We learn about going to bed for colds at an early age. I remember well at the age of seven the glory of staying home from school in bed while watching daytime TV, reading comic books and generally being pampered by my mother with bowls of chicken soup. Unfortunately, bed rest is of no value in treating the symptoms of a cold unless there is significant fever or some other concurrent illness involved. The only person who benefits from your staying at home in bed is the person who would ordinarily sit next to you on the bus or at work. They will probably get it from somebody else anyway.

While you're busy resting in bed, the increased mucous in your airways tends to collect and you may even be increasing your risk of a more serious infection. Getting up and moving around to expand your lungs and keep the cardiovascular system operating at peak efficiency is more likely to help than hurt. The legendary baseball pitcher Satchell Paige recommended getting up and shaking and moving all the limbs from time to time "to keep the juices flowing." This is good advice to anybody with a cold. Of course you shouldn't overdo things. Putting increased demands on your body when it is fighting off the viral assault can tax the system a little too much. I advise patients not to exercise to a point of fatigue or allow themselves to work up a sweat and then get a chill. These can push a simple infection over the edge. Shoveling snow in the cold is not necessarily bad when you have a cold. Shoveling snow and then standing around in your cold wet clothes afterwards is very bad.

When I explain this to patients I often relate two lessons learned during my medical school training. Dr. Louis Weinstein, a pioneer in the field of infectious diseases and one of the true giants of modern medicine, was fond of quoting to his residents and students the words of Benjamin Franklin. Franklin wisely noted that if you doctored a cold it would last a fortnight, and if you didn't, it would last about two weeks. This recognition of the powerlessness of medicine in the face of a common cold is still valid. Most viral colds, from the very first tickle in the throat to the very last cough, will persist from one to two weeks no matter what you do. Often patients will call and say "I'm worried that this cold has lasted so long." I will often respond with Dr. Weinstein's message of patience. The call is most typically prompted by an impending social event, job responsibility or vacation. Usually that's after the third or fourth day.

Another teacher, Dr. Arnold Weinberg, a world reknowned expert in infectious disease and professor at Harvard Medical School regaled his students in the internal medicine board review course many years ago with the words of Dr. William Osler, the father of modern American medicine. Although they are dated in their context, the message is clear. Dr. Osler suggested that when confronted with a common cold, the patient should be advised to go home, put his hat on the bedpost and drink strong whiskey until seeing two hats. This provided fluids, bed rest, cough suppression and calories. Obviously there are problems with this approach, but the overall message remains clear. Science has little to offer in the face of the indomitable common cold. As noted above, sucking on zinc lozenges every two hours will shorten the duration of some cold symptoms by about 48 hours. Faithful adherence to this regimen leaves a foul taste in the mouth and is generally a nuisance. Some are willing to put up with this for the small gain in days of unpleasant stuffiness and congestion, but most people can't sustain the commitment. Except for this option, we don't have any newer or more effective means of treating these particular viral illnesses today than were available more than 200 years ago. Antibiotics, which work against bacterial infections, will not help a viral cold and prescription cough medicines will tend to make you tired and mentally dulled. Though the complications, should they arise, can be managed better, the duration of the basic illness remains unchanged.

Inevitably, a new wave of cold viruses will pass through the community within weeks of the current episode. At this point some will begin to worry why they should have recurrent cold symptoms so soon. Because of all the media hoopla about immunity and terrible infectious diseases, patients become fearful after a second or third viral respiratory illness in a row. One particular group serves as a rich reservoir. School age children, particularly the youngest, tend to touch, feel and slobber all over each other. This keeps respiratory viruses moving around the community. They bring their latest "school project" home and infect their parents who pass it on to friends, family and co-workers. Mothers will often complain, "I've been sick all winter." Though each cold may be relatively mild, the sneezing, coughing and stuffiness are certainly annoying both to the patient and to those who have to listen to the unpleasant sounds they emit. For some, however, this persistent pattern begins to take on the appearance of a dreaded plague or a sign that the system is in trouble. "There must be something wrong. Why do I keep getting sick? Is there something wrong with my immune system?" Some even see these repeat episodes as one long viral illness. They will call day after day wondering and worrying about the ongoing symptoms of a postnasal drip and a drippy nose. I often feel like telling this large group of patients: " Relax. It's not cancer, heart disease, AIDS or the Plague. You will get better eventually and I have nothing in my armamentarium to speed up the process. Be patient and you will recover." I have been known to suggest a trip to the Caribbean as a sure cure. It might not make the virus go away, but it sure will give you something else to think about.

Eventually, the drippy nose and the feeling of mucous in the back of the throat will resolve. If you feel generally well with no fevers, good appetite, plenty of energy and no trouble breathing and all you have is a persistent need to reach for the tissue to blow your nose, then save your time and money and stay away from the doctor's office. It's just a cold.

# *8*

# I CAN'T BELIEVE I ATE THE WHOLE THING: DIGESTIVE DIFFICULTIES

On a recent trip to visit my mother-in-law, my wife and I were awakened at 3 am by her concerned but apologetic voice. She stood at the door to our room with her hands pressed against her breast-bone, belching frequently and complaining that she had severe chest pains. I noted that although she appeared quite fearful, she was breathing normally, not sweating and appeared to be able to walk about the apartment without difficulty. I asked if she was feeling short of breath, which she denied. Knowing that she had a strong heart, few risk factors for heart disease and a negative cardiac exercise test several years earlier, I reminded her of the rather large knockwurst that she had eaten earlier that evening. We discussed briefly the effects of similar dietary indiscretions in the past and then went to the medicine cabinet for some liquid antacid which promptly relieved her symptoms. We sat up and talked for a few minutes until she was sure the problem had resolved and we both returned to sleep. Of course, having a doctor in the house, so to speak, provided a margin of reassurance in this situation. It would have been easy for her to rush to the hospital, dial 911 or call a doctor in the middle of the night.

Many people are fearful of the dire consequences they imagine might occur if they attempt to treat such a problem on their own. They picture the inside of their body, most notably the digestive system, as some mysterious place where strange things happen causing noise and creating foul odors. While there may be some truth to this image, it is fear of the unknown which often triggers the panicked phone call. What if they misdiagnose a heart attack or ignore some feared developing catastrophe which could have been averted? Yet, with a little careful thought, most people could settle a problem like my mother-in-law's without a physician's input. Countless late night emergency room visits and millions of dollars in testing result from a lack of this common sense approach to indigestion, diarrhea, constipation and gas. This is not to say that identical symptoms might not represent an attack of angina or some other vascular emergency. Nor do I suggest that unpleasant bodily symptoms should be ignored. It's just that most indigestion is just that...indigestion.

The events which occur as things move along the gastrointestinal tract can be broken down into ingestion (swallowing), secretion (producing saliva, gastric and intestinal juices and hormones), digestion (breaking down food substances into smaller more usable packets of energy and waste), absorption (getting all the food value from inside of the bowel into the blood stream where it can be used), and excretion (getting rid of what's left over). When problems occur, whether due to illness, stress, diet, medication, or some combination of all of these, they generally occur in one of these basic operations. The terms used most typically are that the symptoms are either functional or organic. Functional symptoms are those which arise from the normal operation of the gastrointestinal system, whereas organic symptoms are caused by sickness or disorder in these operations.

Simple questions need to be asked before rushing off for medical attention. What did I do to provoke this? Have I ever had it before? What did I do to provoke it then and what made it feel better? Do I have any reason to worry about something more serious because of other medical problems or a family history of a related illness? If the answer is obvious and the response to treatment is prompt, don't panic and don't fret. Most important, don't call the doctor, emergency room or Ask a Nurse. On the other hand, if no clear answer can be found, or relief does not follow the previous pattern, or you have real reasons for concern, certainly call for medical attention immediately. However, before putting yourself at the mercy of a medical and surgical diagnostic onslaught, a common sense approach can often avert unnecessary uncomfortable, risky and expensive tests.

The function of the gastrointestinal system should be the easiest for everybody to understand. You put something in one end, it moves along a tube as things happen to it and what's left comes out the other end. This ought to be pretty simple stuff. In spite of this, most people are unwilling or unable to understand that what you put in will affect what comes out. For those who remember the advertisements of 25 years ago, the response of the digestive system can be summarized by the ad campaign for an antacid which shows a man leaning over his plate exclaiming "Mama mia! Atsa some spicy meatballs!" Follow this with the ad from the same company which has a distressed looking individual looking at an empty plate moaning "I can't believe I ate the whole thing."

It's so obvious. The average person can recognize easily that if you buy gasoline for your car at a location which is not your custom and an hour or two later it starts skipping and smoking and stalling (nausea, belching and constipaton), the cause is likely to be the gasoline, not the car. The likely decision would be to avoid putting that particular gasoline into the car again out of fear it would cause damage. The noise and smoke and interrupted locomotion would be at the least, a nuisance. Yet the same person will repeatedly ingest the hot salsa and beer which has given him indigestion, gas and cramps on many earlier occasions. He may or may not make the cause and effect connection, and yet will continue to perform the same behavior pattern.

Cheryl is a 38 year old mother of two children under the age of 10. Her husband is a non-communicative, hard working businessman who has had a series of financial successes and reverses over the past ten years. The couple's material success has not achieved the level expected by my patient's mother who makes her aware of this on a regular basis. Throughout the duration of the marriage, Cheryl has seen me frequently for symptoms of heartburn, indigestion, stomach cramps, constipation, diarrhea, nausea and gas. As we treat each new problem, another develops. She has been consistently unable to connect her life situation with her symptoms in spite of an array of normal laboratory tests, x-rays and other diagnostic studies that would choke most insurance companies. Most of our meetings start off discussing her latest complaint, but end up with her in tears, relating the latest family turmoil. I offer counseling and advice, suggest marital therapy, and, when pressed, perhaps a new medication for her complaints. On rare occasions she has wondered about the effect of stress on her symptoms and I revel at the prospect of addressing the real cause of her problems. She has even agreed to a few visits with a social worker and a psychologist. In spite of these brief breakthroughs, she continues to return and call every week with the latest presentation of her gastrointestinal difficulties.

The technical term for Cheryl's problem is Irritable Bowel Syndrome which most often presents as a constant barrage of gastrointestinal symptoms often alternating between opposing malfunctions (diarrhea and constipation, gas and bloating) occurring over many years and not associated with any evidence of progressive disease. The symptoms are often made worse at times of stress or anxiety or in association with poor dietary habits. These are not the patients who come in with six weeks of new symptoms, but rather those who recall symptoms going back to high school with long periods of feeling well in between. It is not at all uncommon for people with these difficulties to undergo all the various diagnostic procedures on multiple occasions in the vain hope that they will find a simple explanation and cure. Some may actually turn out to have some medical disorder that requires treatment, though most do not. Out of frustration, they will often pass from doctor to doctor looking for the one who will solve the riddle. Over time, however, good physicians try to educate patients to understand the diagnosis and the options for treatment. Hopefully, by accepting the occasional cramp and disordered bowel function, they will recognize the symptoms which occur in response to some environmental challenge such as a stressful day at home or at work, an overdose of salsa or barbecue delights, sleeplessness for whatever reason, or an overly large meal at cousin Emily's wedding.

Probably the most common gastrointestinal complaint is excessive gas. People seem to have trouble accepting that gas, whether belching or flatus, is a normal product of the digestive tract. It is the result of gas production during the process of breakdown of food substances. Some foods generate more gas than others. Everybody knows about beans, immortalized in the movie Blazing Saddles. As a child I remember my father singing the ditty he learned in the army about "beans, beans, the musical fruit." Interestingly enough, many of the foods which we have all learned to take for granted as healthy have a tremendous potential to be a source of gas such as cruciferous vegetables like cabbage, broccoli, cauliflower, and lettuce, complex carbohydrates such as pasta and breads (particularly bagels), and of course beans. Though it may be socially embarrassing and aesthetically unpleasant, particularly in a crowded elevator, the expulsion of gas is a natural and healthy phenomenon. It is more a function of gastronomic preference than bowel normality. Sometimes gas can be produced by malfunctioning intestines, as in lactose intolerance, the inability to digest milk sugar. For this reason, most physicians will advise patients with this complaint to avoid all dairy products for a few weeks. If the symptoms go away and return when you resume dairy products again, then you have a diagnosis and treatment. You don't need any special tests or doctors.

Occasionally gas results from constipation due to a diet deficient in fiber and liquid. Often adding a few tablespoons of unprocessed bran or bran cereal along with adequate amounts of liquid each day (at least the equivalent of four 8 oz glasses of water) will correct the problem. Of course, the liquid should not be carbonated. Beverages of this sort get their fizz from carbon dioxide gas dissolved at low temperatures in the liquid. When it is heated up, either sitting out in the sun or inside your warm stomach, the gas is released and must go somewhere. If you're having a few cans of soda in some form each day, expect gas. Or consider switching to water. After trying all the above remedies, if you still feel gassy, make an appointment to see your doctor, but don't be disappointed if no firm diagnosis or treatment is offered. There may be none necessary. At the same time, beware of overzealous medical care. Be certain you are convinced of your symptoms because they will likely be taken seriously.

Gastrointestinal complaints are the bread and butter of most medical practices and provide a rich source of income to the pharmaceutical industry. Burping, belching, flatus, constipation, diarrhea, indigestion, heartburn, hemerrhoids. There's enough to keep any physician busy and generate a lifetime of work, though, in truth, most sufferers require no medical attention. I know many physicians who are happy to see patients with these complaints over and over again in spite of normal tests while clearly understanding they have little to offer in the way of scientific treatment. Rather than tell these patients that they should stop worrying, eat properly and take over the counter medicines when problems act up, they often repeatedly run the patients through expensive and sometimes risky tests. Specialists feel a particular need to give people their money's worth and are a frequent source of this disease-oriented approach to complaints. Large multispecialty clinics across the country are notorious for this aggressive, illness oriented, test for everything approach with no evidence that their patients live longer, healthier or better. Their methods are consistent with our traditional medical training which assumes that a person requesting medical attention is sick rather than assuming they are well. This only serves to reinforce the patient's belief that he suffers a medical illness and feeds his need for more costly medical attention. At the same time it weakens his sense of wholeness or integrity.

I am reminded of Sal, a hard working, driven and incredibly anxious 34 year old father of two little boys. When his anxiety gets out of control, he has diarrhea for a day or two. He blames this on the food he has recently eaten and his digestive tract. Often he will avoid eating because he feels it triggers his symptoms. Over time, his therapist and I have helped him to connect his anxiety with his symptoms and accept his own basic good health. He appeared to be improving with a combination of counseling and occasional medication when, at the recommendation of a friend, he went to see a prominent gastroenterologist in town. As expected, he underwent an upper and lower gastrointestinal x-ray series, followed by a sigmoidoscopy. I knew he would find the latter procedure unbearable because of his fastidious nature, but there was nothing I could do to prevent it. I'm sure he knew I would not approve of all the testing since he failed to apprise me of the plan until after he had finished. The final diagnosis was functional bowel disease, as I expected. Now, rather than send Sal back to his therapist and his primary care physician, the specialist continues to see him on a regular basis for his non-disease. Sal now views his symptoms as part of a disease syndrome and the subspecialist is a little busier and a little richer.

Because we continuously use our intestines, some patients manage to complain of just about every gastrointestinal symptom at one time or another. Norman, a patient who I have seen for more than fifteen years will call on Monday complaining of diarrhea and cramps, then call back two days later with a feeling of constipation and bloating. No matter which, he always has pains and cramping. In spite of the fact that these symptoms have been unchanged for over a decade and a half and after several extensive medical evaluations, he remains convinced that we are missing some ghastly illness. He will often go to see another of the many specialists he has visited over the years who will promptly run a new series of tests. Nothing new is found, yet he adds these doctors to his long list of consultants. Recently, in spite of my reassurances that his breathlessness and chest discomfort after meals was due to his obesity and poor dietary habits, he visited a cardiologist who sent him off for an angiogram which, of course, was fine. When I called him before the test he asked if I thought he was taking an unnecessary risk. I did not want to create fear and uncertainty prior to the study. I reassured him that I thought all would go well. He told me of his worry that we might be missing something. Once again, as expected, the test was normal.

This pattern is not at all uncommon to physicians who treat general medical patients. While he focuses on fluctuations in normal bodily functions such as belching, passing flatus, and an occasional abdominal cramp, the complaint is in reality an expression of his emotional distress. Norman is unable to recognize the chronic and repetitive nature of his symptoms. In spite of our often lengthy discussions regarding business reverses and troubled family relationships, he seems unable to connect these issues with his fear of physical discomfort.

I am often struck by the willingness of my colleagues to play into this fear and anxiety. They do so for several reasons. Some believe they truly know more than all the previous specialists and internists and can solve the patient's complaint by virtue of their own brilliance. While this may be true on occasion, more often it is not. This attitude feeds the already substantial ego of the average physician who is asked to reevaluate somebody who has only recently come through the medical diagnostic machine. Since failure to make a diagnosis is a common reason for malpractice lawsuits, some doctors feel compelled to repeat all previously performed studies and extend the evaluation in order to avoid the risk of litigation. Still others run tests which will bring them financial rewards because of their ability to order tests on lucrative equipment they control, such as laboratory and xray machines, heart testing facilities and endoscopy. Overall, they leave the patient dependent on their role as a specialist, while at the same time taking a medically well patient and allowing him to view himself as a victim of disease.

A college student whom I have seen since her early adolescent days came in recently with her usual complaints of stomach cramps and diarrhea only this time it was worse. Nothing in her life was different, she insisted. There were no new stresses and she was generally happy. As I explored the history of her symptoms it became apparent that she was having spells like this two or three times a week.

"Let's review your diet for the past 48 hours," I suggested. She had little to reveal, eating a reasonably healthy series of meals.

"Nothing else?" I queried.

"Well, I did have several gin and tonics two nights ago."

"Several?"

"You know. Five or six."

"How many times a week does this occur."

I suppose I should have been prepared for her response of two or three times week. Yet knowing how long we had dealt with her gastrointestinal difficulties, I found myself a little stunned. In the best non-judgemental tone I could muster, I explained that not only was the poisoning of her gastrointestinal tract the likely direct cause of her current problems, the volume and frequency of her alcohol intake concerned me deeply. We talked about this for some time and I believe she understood finally the relationship between her symptoms and her alcohol abuse. Like many, however, I wasn't convinced she would change her habit immediatly..

It's not fair for me to be overly critical here. Like the majority of

American Jews and African Americans, I suffer from an inability to fully digest foods containing milk, a disorder commonly known as lactose intolerance. This is due to an inherited deficiency of the enzyme lactase which breaks down lactose, the major sugar found in milk. When lactose is not digested properly it passes into the large intestine where it is acted upon by bacteria commonly found there. This leads to the formation of gas and digestive by-products which gives way to bloating, distention, cramping and occasionally diarrhea. In spite of this I will on occasion consume a creamed soup, a dairy queen cone or have a sandwich with cheese, knowing well the unpleasant consequences which will inevitably follow. When was the last time you looked at something to eat and thought, "I know I'll regret it, but it looks so good. How can I resist? I'll have it just this once." I know I have done this, and I have paid the price with distress and unpleasant gastrointestinal symptoms.

Unfortunately, the piper must be paid at some point. Abuse of the gastrointestinal tract will lead to unpleasant symptoms. We all forget too easily that our body and its normal functioning is a gift. Like most gifts, however, maintenance and upkeep is our responsibility. The important message is that our bodies have a remarkable ability to recover from our abuse if we just let up on the indiscretion. We control whether or not the problem occurs and clearly understand the cause and treatment without the services of the medical profession. Most symptoms usually can be managed with rest and time. If you can't stand it, over the counter preparations can be used with good response-antacid for heartburn, antacid with simethicone for heartburn and gas, anti-diarrheal agents or chamomile tea and boiled rice when needed to control symptoms that last more than 12 hours or that interfere with your activities. However, just as all these treatments indicate on the box, be wary of symptoms that worsen, don't respond or last more than 48 hours. Then it's time to call the doctor. Don't panic. Don't rush to the emergency room or call on the services of a medical specialist. Simply review the problem with your internist or family practitioner.

Often I find myself silently observing patients as they relate to me their various types of abdominal symptoms for which they appear to have no explanation and about which they fear the very worst is about to happen- that I will tell them they clearly have some horrible fatal disorder. I then ask them to describe to me all the awful things they swallowed in the previous day, week, month or year as well as the nature of any unusual stresses at home or at work. Even the most stubborn will eventually begin to make some meaningful association between their diet, stress and symptoms, though it often takes many tests, medications and occasionally other opinions for acceptance to occur.

One woman I follow has undergone repeated upper gastrointestinal x-rays, endoscopies (the passage of a tube down through the throat into the esophagus and stomach and looking around through the benefit of fiberoptics), biopsies and even a rather substantial surgical procedure to try to reduce the amount of acid washing up from her stomach into her esophagus. Yet she continues to come in complaining of chronic heartburn and denies any association with her dietary intake. No matter how hard I have pressed in an effort to find the clue to her ongoing problems, I was uniformly unsuccessful. Imagine my surprise when I passed her at a restaurant table where she was consuming a large serving of Cippino, a highly spiced seafood somewhat akin to bouillabaisse, and washing it down with what appeared to be liberal amounts of a fine wine. I said hello simply to let her know that I was a witness, but did not mention the association until her next visit which of course followed shortly afterwards. For a year she complained less frequently and seemed to accept her culpability in perpetuating the problem. It seems, however, that memory is short, and she resumed her errant ways.

This is not to deny that the same symptoms might be a harbinger of something worse. However, there tends to be a qualitative difference in that setting. Either there is no warning and a tumor or disease appears without any detectable sign, or the presenting symptoms develop insidiously but progressively over a distinguishable period of time. Somebody with constipation and cramping for ten years doesn't have a new colon cancer because those symptoms were present. It is pure coincidence and no association can be made. On the other hand, if that same patient notes a gradual but progressive change in the character of the bowel movements for more than a few weeks, that would be worthy of note. A sharp pain in the abdomen that doesn't take your breath away and lasts only a few seconds but does not recur is probably nothing to worry about. When a patient tells me they have pain in the abdomen for a minute after every meal for 15 years, I tell them to be sure to call me when the pain goes away. If the same pain starts coming on every day or every other day and lasts longer and longer or if you notice a pattern to the pain in association with meals or bowel movements, then we have a potential problem. The difference in the way these problems present sends a clear message that I repeat to my patients as often as necessary. Don't worry about things that go away.

Everybody needs to understand his body's reactions. Don't be alarmed at minor transient disturbances. We are not designed by our Creator to mechanically march along without some reaction to the forces around us. Thank goodness our stomachs will expel noxious substances which can cause it harm. Thank goodness the distention of our bellys from overeating or the overindulgence of alcohol send us clear signals with pain, belching and distention, warning us that we need to change our ways. Thank goodness our intestines can warn us when we are letting stress hurt us inside. Rather than fear disease from our gastrointestinal system, we need to recognize its responses and listen to the messages. We can rush off to the doctor for every cramp or belch or we can choose to think through the problem and try to deal with it.

# *9*

## MEDICINES AND TREATMENTS: THE GOOD NEWS AND THE BAD NEWS

Helen is a 47 year old woman who weighs 260 pounds and stands 5 feet tall in her stocking feet. Over the years I have watched her develop diabetes, high blood pressure, gout and arthritis in her knees and hips from carrying her prodigious frame from place to place. As each new problem developed, she repeatedly rejected attempts to use medication to prevent her difficulties or control the potential complications from them. Each time she knew all the right questions, primed by the latest health letter or news item. Often we would debate for months the need and safety of various medications, until, convinced of the ultimate benefit of control and the relative safety of the drug, she would relent. The blood pressure medicine might make her depressed, dull her sexual drive, interfere with her sleep pattern or cause her to cough. She read that it might cause her to become constipated or even worse, cause cancer.

It was a constant chore to keep her on medication for her gout. She had read in her home medical consumer guide about the risks of the drug and its potential to affect her liver or her blood counts. My efforts to explain the possible damage the disorder could cause to her kidneys and joints were to no avail. She asked if there were some herbal or homeopathic remedy. She was willing to do almost anything but take a prescribed medication. However, enough painful attacks of gout convinced her. When it came to managing her diabetes, she swore month after month that she would achieve control with a better diet and more exercise, though we both knew this would never happen. The problem was exacerbated by memories of her mother's death from diabetes. She saw her mother's treatment with pills and insulin as the cause of her slow and unpleasant end, rather than recognizing that the deterioration was due to a similar unwillingness to comply with her medical management as well as the natural course of the illness in its advanced stages.

With all this fear and avoidance of medication, imagine my surprise when she came in asking for the newly publicized diet pill combination as a cure to her problems. She was convinced that simply taking these pills would eliminate her difficulties in life. Though I recognized the connection between her body image and her desperate willingness to try something new, I was puzzled by her eagerness to try a treatment which was new and potentially dangerous, given her avoidance of well established medical treatments in the past. I pointed out that it was one thing to show a drug's safety in a trial of 20,000 patients, but quite another to know what would happen after millions of people began taking these drugs. Under much pressure and after several visits and several months delay, I acquiesced and initiated treatment with the medications. Within a short period of time it became apparent that not only was the medicine not working, but it was also giving her unacceptable side effects with severe constipation and daytime sleepiness. At the same time, new research indicated more dangers from use of this treatment. We stopped the drugs. She viewed this as another sign of her failure and a confirmation of her belief that all medicine is basically bad for her.

Helen's story, a common occurrence in most medical practices, summarizes the critical problems I face with patients when attempting to address the issue of medications:

1.  Caution to the point of undue suspicion
2.  Unrealistic expectations
3.  Excessive reliance on the media rather than physicians and pharmacists as a source of information
4.  Abuse of medications by patients and physicians
5.  Lack of basic trust

A striking dichotomy exists between the desire for treatment and the need to avoid medication. Like Helen, many patients delay necessary medication out of an understandable but often irrational fear of the possible dangers. This is often supported by horror stories they have read or heard, that medications are basically dangerous and likely to do them more harm than good.

The classic example of this behavior with which most primary care physicians are familiar is the asthmatic patient who constantly tries to stop or "forget to take" medications. In a subconscious effort to deny the disease, deny their fallibility, this group of patients is notorious for trying to get off medications which are critical to their health. It is easy to understand why a person with asthma wants to avoid pulling out his plastic medication inhaler in public or even in front of his spouse or partner. There is a clear need to hide the difficulty from others and from themselves. Those who suffer from asthma often have difficulty acknowledging in their own minds the need to depend on medication. It implies a sense of being somehow less than whole, less in control of oneself. It creates a feeling of being not normal. When a patient says to me "Why do I have to do this?" it is not for lack of understanding the diagnosis and action of the medication which I have already explained in detail. Rather, the question arises from a more existential pain asking "Why is this happening to me?"

These patients, like most of us, view the need for medication as an affront to their sense of wholeness. Fear of or unwillingness to take medications stems from a basic need for constant reaffirmation of youth and fitness which in its essence arises from a fear of death and pain. Medication symbolizes for many aging, infirmity, pain and death rather than healing and wellness. When you are feeling well, identification with this unpleasant image often stands in the way of taking medication which might have the potential for prolonging and improving the quality of life.

A particular patient comes to mind in this setting. This pleasant 39 year old woman had delivered her first child only six months earlier which, because of her age, was a particularly strong source of personal fulfillment. She complained of the usual post partum difficulty with weight gain and fatigue, but minimized her complaints in deference to her joy over the new baby, whose pictures she laid out for me to view. Only those who have experienced or been intimately involved in a prolonged period of infertility and childlessness can appreciate the effervescence of her joy. Although I was happy for her, having participated in the many years of diagnostic tests, treatments and emotional turmoil, I needed to tell her that her examination and symptoms suggested that she had an underactive thyroid. I pointed out that this was very common after pregnancy and often resolved spontaneously. I provided what I thought was lots of reassurance regarding the minor nature of this problem and the lack of impact it would have on her life. When I told her she would need to take thyroid replacement pills for an as yet indeterminate period of time, she looked as though I was about to take her child away. In truth, I was taking from her part of this newly found sense of being a complete person she had found through the birth of her child. She accepted the treatment with a surprising stoicism, which I thought was uncharacteristic.

During the ensuing ten weeks, while I waited to repeat her blood test to measure the effectiveness of the treatment, I did not hear from her at all. When she returned, again with more pictures of the growing child, along with stories of the daughter's spectacular achievements, she denied any symptoms of fatigue or other signs of illness. I was puzzled to find that her laboratory tests indicated inadequate replacement levels of thyroid hormone. While this often happens with initial attempts to estimate the correct dose of medication, I was frustrated repeatedly with subsequent tests, in spite of increasing doses of the medication.

After five months of this, I decided to confront her with my suspicions, particularly as she began to show clinical evidence of the effect of inadequate thyroid hormone. After once again viewing the latest collection of pictures and hearing the latest stories of the child's successes, I asked her to tell me honestly whether or not she was actually taking the medication as prescribed in spite of having told me previously that she had not missed any. She flushed and began fiddling with her pictures, and with a quivering voice, admitted that she often missed taking them up to five or six times a week and in fact had not taken any in over a month. I honestly tried not to be a stern parent figure as I stared rather blankly at her. I then re-iterated the potential dangers she faced if she had significantly diminished thyroid activity which remained untreated.

She has been better since then, but still lapses into periods of not taking her medications regularly. The comical twist in the story came when she brought her mother in for her routine visit and I found that her blood pressure medication had appeared to lose it's effect. This often happens, particularly in the elderly. In this setting, blood pressure medicine requires changes and adjustments. I wasn't alarmed until her daughter, the recalcitrant taker of thyroid, piped in with a chastisement that nearly floored me. "You're not telling the doctor the whole story, mother. You know perfectly well that you don't like to take your medicines and miss the blood pressure pills most of the time." I quickly interjected, half in jest, "like mother, like daughter." The mother looked at me quizzically, and the daughter looked at me as if I were on another planet. Somehow, neither could acknowledge their unwillingness to accept the need for medication.

Often patients will appropriately ask, "How will this hurt me? What are the risks?" "Will I get hooked on this? I don't want to become dependent on anything." Certainly it's important to ask about potential medication side effects and risks. One needs to check for any potential adverse interactions between drugs. However, the issue of dependence is much maligned. When medical professionals discuss drug dependence, we mean a situation involving a physical need for medication which increases over time and which provides a response in the patient which is other than that intended when the medication was originally prescribed. For example, morphine is given for pain relief, usually in the setting of severe injury such as a burn, or in the post operative state.

Dependency occurs when the patient's goal in taking the medication is to regain a state of bodily or mental sensation unrelated to the original use of the drug. In dependency, the body requires ever increasing amounts of the medication to quench the desire. This phenomenon is very different from the patient with high blood pressure, asthma, diabetes, arthritis or other chronic illness. In that setting, the medication relieves a symptom or manifestation of a disease. Because it works, often the patient feels better, or at least recognizes a real benefit from the drug. The medicine is continued for the sake of that improved medical state and occasional sense of well being. In a way, there is a dependence. Without the medication the body will get back into the original trouble. However, unlike the situation with a true addicting drug, the treatment can be stopped at any time with no residual craving or desire to take the pills.

So you shouldn't worry about getting hooked on your blood pressure pills or dependent on your asthma, thyroid or heart medicines. Take them because you need them to stay well.

I understand clearly the desire to avoid dependence on medication. Taking pills is the existential equivalent of saying "I'm not whole. I'm fallible. In order to function, I must take this artificial substance. My life and my happiness are now dependent on putting a manufactured substance into my body. Who knows what this could lead to with side effects and all the problems with chemicals." These are natural responses to the diagnosis of a medical condition. We all would like to feel whole, healthy and perfect, or at least something approaching perfect. Nearly everybody wants to leave the office having been told they are in good health with no medical problems. That's why going to the doctor's office is such a threat in the first place. Unfortunately, life is not perfect and illness and medical conditions occur. Much of the popular focus on natural approaches to healing comes out of this desire to avoid medication, but even more out of an unwillingness to accept human vulnerability and a lack of control. Taking medication is often perceived as relinquishing control to some faceless corporate entity churning out pills and capsules by the millions with no attachment to the sick patient. How could they possibly know about the individuals needs and problems? Helping patients to accept the physician's role as an intermediary in this process without turning it into an existential crisis is one of the hardest parts of my job. Resistance to diagnosis and treatment of medical conditions is legendary and can be almost comical.

Here's the scene: Mr. Smith is sitting across from me at my desk. He is swarthy complected, mildly over weight, with the broad hands of one who is used to hard physical labor.

"Mr. Smith, your blood pressure is dangerously high, and I want to prevent it from causing a stroke, heart attack or kidney failure. If you take this medicine once a day, it should control the pressure and prevent any of these serious problems. Medical research has shown that treating high blood pressure with medications can significantly prolong and improve the quality of life. You may have some mild side effects such as (this will vary according to the type of medication), but I have a lot of experience with this medication and I believe it is safe for you to try. Besides, the side effects are not common and, in any event, we can always stop the medication."

"Well, I suppose I should" he replies, clearly a little tentative, "but I hear these medicines can be dangerous. I don't like to put chemicals into my body." That seems to be a watchword. Chemicals. Anything made by a drug company is a chemical and therefore dangerous.

"I understand. Unfortunately we've tried dieting and exercise as well as the meditation course you took, and they don't seem to have helped. Now you sit here with this significant high blood pressure and I'm a little concerned about leaving it untreated. At this point, the risk of high blood pressure to your health and survival is far greater than the potential risk of this or most medications."

"Well, do you think I should get another opinion?"

"You're welcome to get all the opinions you want. I assume you came to see me because you trust my judgment. My judgment is that you need to treat this problem. I can assure you that anybody suggesting that you not take medications is giving you bad advice. I can also assure you that I would not give you any medication if I thought the risk of the medication was significant and particularly if I did not feel on balance that the benefits far outweighed the risks." This fear and suspicion is not a new phenomenon. My grandfather who died several years ago at 94 never liked taking his medication, and he was always suspicious of any new prescription. But when his doctor firmly told him he needed to take something, he did.

We are obsessed with medications, both in a positive and negative sense. This obsession intrudes into our lives on a daily basis, both with regard to dealing with ordinary problems like colds, bladder infections and acne, and also in dealing with more complex medical issues such as high blood pressure, diabetes, pregnancy and cancer, to name just a few. In order to overcome this, we need to understand and accept a few basic assumptions with regard to medicine, medical care and drugs.

In general, advancements in science and medicine have served to improve the quality and length of life. The average life expectancy of an American citizen has improved dramatically over the course of the modern scientific era from 49 years at the turn of the century to 76 years at the end of this century. Although much of this has resulted from public health measures such as improved public sanitation and water supplies, a large part of it has also resulted from the use of medications that eliminated or controlled common diseases which were the scourge of the earlier time. With the advent of penicillin in the early 1940's, many infectious diseases which led to early death and disability were controlled. My wife's grandfather who died in 1941 of an infection of his heart valve at the age of 44, might have lived to see his children and great grandchildren had he been fortunate to have lived just a few short months until penicillin was commonly available. On the other hand, her grandmother, a delightful woman who suffered from chronic congestive heart failure and diabetes, lived many years beyond her expected survival due to the benefits from some of the newer drugs available for treating this disorder.

High blood pressure, a common disorder affecting over 30 million Americans, is one of the most common causes of stroke and kidney failure. The cost to our economy and national productivity of untreated high blood pressure has been estimated in the many billions of dollars each year. More important, the pain and suffering experienced by these many millions of people leaves a devastating scar on our national soul. All the data collected over the many years during which good treatment for high blood pressure has been available indicate that the use of medication to control this problem clearly and unequivocally leads to improvement in the quality and prolongation of life. This evidence holds true even if one takes into account the potential for side effects of these medications. New and accumulating evidence indicates that some medicines for elevated cholesterol can reduce the risk of early heart attack and prevent progression of pre-existing coronary disease. Some studies even show that people live longer and more productively with these medicines. Polio, a scourge in this country only 45 years ago and a continued health problem around the world has been eliminated as a serious illness in the United States due to an aggressive program of vaccination. We now have within our reach the ability to nearly eliminate all new cases of measles, german measles, mumps, diphtheria, tetanus and hepatitis A and B. Influenza, a common cause of death in the elderly and chronically ill, can be prevented or at least decreased in severity by the seasonal use of influenza vaccine. All this depends on a willingness to commit national resources to the goal and more important, a willingness to accept the vaccines.

An interesting side note is that, while most managed care plans encourage prevention as a marketing tool, they make it very difficult for patients or physicians to be compensated for the cost of vaccines. This is because reducing disease is a long-term goal while paying for expensive vaccines hurts the bottom line of the corporate balance sheet. So we have the tools and the skills to prevent illness, and yet, in the community we are met by tremendous resistance to treatment.

A reasonable person might ask at this point, with all the drugs and all the diseases medicine must face, how can you be sure you can trust your doctors about taking or not taking medicines. In spite of all you may read about careless doctors and malpractice, most doctors are well trained and honestly interested in your well-being. They don't get kickbacks from drug companies or pharmacies and their only interest in treating you is to make you well or to keep you from getting sick. A good way to test this is by observing your doctor's response to any questions or suggestions you might have. If you mention that your Aunt Sara is on a particular drug for her blood pressure and it seems to work well for her, your doctor should be able to respond with reasons not to chose that particular medication or at least a willingness to consider it as an option. If the response is satisfactory, then you should try to trust this person in whose hands you are placing your life. If, on the other hand, the response is defensive or hostile, you need to question if the doctor considers his or her ego or some other source of reward as more significant than your needs or interests.

Trust must exist at some point between you and your physician so that you don't need to worry constantly, in spite of the media's warnings. A constant state of suspicion is not conducive to a working relationship with your doctor. I have seen patients unnecessarily delay beginning treatment for dangerously long periods of time, believing either that the problem will go away or that the medication is worse than the problem. They usually bring in articles from magazines and newspapers and copies of the appropriate section from the PDR (physician's desk reference) with a long list of potential problems. I thank them for the information, assuring them that I will look into the matter, if I am indeed unaware. At the same time, I try to instill a feeling of trust that I will keep their best interest at heart. It is this sense of trust between patient and doctor which has suffered so much under the consumerist onslaught of our commercial culture. Though most professionals are honest and deserving of trust, it is the extremes which cause a feeling of alarm. And, of course, it is the extremes that sell newspapers and improve viewership for the media. Between dishonest lawyers, pedophilic clergy, abusive policemen, and sexually deviant and greedy physicians, it's easy to understand why patients would be suspicious of any person in authority. By raising doubts and fears about physician behavior and medications, the print and electronic media flame the fire of uncertainty about diagnosis and treatments. This encourages a sense of excessive reliance on the media rather than on physicians and pharmacists as the source of information about medications. This unfortunately works in opposing directions, encouraging pursuit of the latest drug to be released at the same time as patients are chastised to avoid overmedication.

Your doctor may tell you that in spite of your efforts or lack of them to reduce weight and exercise aerobically, you still need to take medication for high blood pressure. Or you might be told you need thyroid replacement to correct an imbalance in your body. Perhaps you might be encouraged to take a medication to prevent black out spells or heart rhythm problems. Ask about the risks and side effects. Be certain you understand the reason for taking the medication and the method for measuring its action. Consider the potential value of treating versus not treating. Remember, though, that your doctor wants you to be well and live long. Unless the arguments not to treat still seem strong, listen to the advice of your doctor. If you don't trust your doctor, get another medical opinion. But don't neglect the problem. Ultimately its your choice.

# *10*

## EYE OF NEWT AND TOE OF FROG: HERBS AND VITAMINS

As my wife and I enjoyed breakfast one perfect morning, sitting at the edge of a Caribbean beach, I watched a plump woman of about 60 finish her croissant, coffee, cereal and fruit, and then pull out a plastic bag. From this she extracted 8 smaller neatly labeled bags containing what by my discerning eye were a colorful assortment of vitamins, herbal compounds, minerals and bowel stimulants. She carefully placed them together on the table before her. Other similar collections remained in the larger bag, obviously to be taken at some other time of day. Her husband looked on in what appeared to be a distant and possibly disapproving manner, though I may have been projecting the latter. She re-checked her count and labels, presumably to be certain she hadn't missed any, and then proceeded to wash them down with good French coffee-her second cup by my count.

It's important to appreciate the setting in order to understand this behavior. The island we were visiting had perfect weather, perfect beaches, perfect food, beautiful people, no crime and no apparent poverty. If it weren't so expensive, it would be something close to paradise. For most of us a visit is something that happens because you've managed to save enough frequent flier miles and are willing to accept the debt. For others, it might be a stopover on a bargain holiday cruise. But for this couple, it was clear the cost of the visit was no financial strain. She wore subtle but expensive jewelry, perfect make-up and just the right clothes. Here she sat in near paradise. Rather than sitting back and taking in the beautiful blue water and sky, verdant rolling hills, white sand beach and gentle breeze, her most important concern was getting into her body all these things that somebody convinced her would prolong her life, make her young again or give her energy. Some so-called holistic doctor or self-proclaimed herbal specialist had her convinced that these supplements were necessary.

I felt an urge to approach her, turn her to the ocean and say gently, lady, this is life. Take it in. Breathe it. Smell it. Feel it. Whatever is bothering you, go out and stand on the beach and say to the wind, "I can see. I can hear. I can walk. My body performs its normal functions. Nobody is trying to kill me, take away my home, abuse my children. Look at this setting. Look at this place. How lucky I am to be alive on this magnificent day." Since I was on vacation I figured my wife would probably kill me if I even spoke to her, let alone confront her in such a dramatic manner, so I kept my peace.

I am amazed at the numbers of patients who come to see me with exactly this story. Whether they come with complaints or not, they will list an array of herbs, potions, powders and concoctions that they are daily putting into their systems. They gather information from tabloids at the supermarket check-out stands, clerks working in health food stores, friends at work or in social settings, magazines capitalizing on the enormous market, the internet and self appointed fitness experts at gyms and spas, many of whom receive fees and benefits for promoting particular brands. I find it truly remarkable that a patient will question the risks of a cholesterol lowering pill, blood pressure medicine or antibiotic when offered by a physician but will readily accept some mysterious concoction from almost anybody if it's called natural or an herb. I sometimes feel it would be easier to get some patients to take their medication if I called it a tonic or potion purchased through a pharmacist who dressed in appropriate costume and called herself a medicine man.

One 67 year old man in general good health gave me a list including apple pectin, garlic, vitamin C, zinc, lecithin, blue green algae, echanacia, gingko biloba, and coenzyme Q10. As is often the case, I found myself scratching my head with what I assume was a somewhat incredulous expression on my face. "Why on earth are you taking all this stuff?" I asked. His response was characteristic of patients who have bought into the whole scene. "Don't you believe in vitamins and natural holistic remedies?"

The answer is a complicated yes and no. It's not that I don't recognize the utility of many herbs and some supplements. Every morning I take a multivitamin and 400 units of vitamin E. I would also take a small dose of aspirin if I hadn't found that it upset my stomach. I understand the feeling of helplessness created by the fear of illness and fostered by the medical profession and need to assert a sense of control over one's fate. I'm just a natural born skeptic about most things. This is the result of appreciating the importance of the scientific method and the need for proof in moving civilization out of the dark ages. It also came from listening to my grandmother who taught me at a very early age to believe none of what I hear and only half of what I see. So when a patient asks if I believe in vitamins, I explain that belief is a strong word which I reserve for matters that have been proven beyond a reasonable doubt or those questions which require religious commitment and are to be taken on faith. I understand clearly the difference between faith and belief.

For many people, unfortunately, uncritical blind acceptance of vitamins and so called natural and holistic remedies to bring health and create a feeling of control has achieved the level of religious fervor. Don't be confused by the lack of scientific proof or the unknown potential risks. If it's holistic and it's natural, it must be good. Often proponents will cite the work of a medical research lab, sometimes even at respected university, as "proof" of support by the scientific community. This naive approach to scientific research fails to recognize that very little is accepted as proven by the scientific community until it has been critically reviewed and duplicated in other laboratories. People suffering from disabling and terminal illnesses for whom traditional medicine has limited options will reach out to anything that promises hope. Countless patients, including members of my own family, when faced with the diagnosis of cancer or the pain and disability of chronic disease choose this option. They are vulnerable to merchants of all sorts and motivations offering ostensible cures or treatments. Often attempts to promote a treatment, because of purported success in a handful of scattered patients, fall apart when the study is scrutinized to look for other factors which might influence the study result.

One of the most difficult tasks I've faced in all my years in medicine was the day I had to sit down with a couple who are among my oldest and dearest friends to deliver some painful news. I had just finished reviewing the laboratory results of their daughter, Rachel, whom I had known since early childhood and who had just graduated from college. With a heavy heart, I explained that she had developed acute myelogenous leukemia. After the initial shock, Rachel faced down the illness and valiantly made it through a successful bone marrow transplant. After months of weakness, fevers, pain, deprivation of a sense of self and a year of isolation, she recovered. I still savor the day when she leaped off my sailboat into the ocean off of Martha's Vineyard on her first day of returning to the real world. She was back, and we rejoiced in the moment.

Sadly, 18 months later she had the incredible misfortune of relapsing with her original leukemia. As we all agonized through the decision process as to where to go next with her treatment, Rachel decided to assert some control over her treatment. She elected to put off her repeat transplant, which we all saw as a step back into the levels of hell, and try a course of an herbal remedy known as Essiac. The medical community has looked at this and found it to be a relatively harmless mixture of things that have been coincidentally associated with favorable outcomes in some patients. There is, however, no reliable scientific evidence that it really does anything at all.

When her father asked me if I thought there would be anything wrong with this course, I reassured him that we had no immediate need to rush into her chemotherapy. If she wanted to do this for a while, if it would give her a sense of control, then why not? I was willing to try anything, to hope for a miracle for somebody in such desperate straits, if there was nothing to lose. I did not for one minute expect her to benefit from this treatment. As we discussed the potential benefits and risks, he reassured me that there could be no downside since these were herbs and not chemicals. This is a misconception of such enormous proportions that I have to pause and collect myself when I hear it spoken. It asserts a desire to believe that medicines of the traditional type are chemicals and therefore bad and that herbs are natural, not chemicals, and therefore good. I tried to point out to Rachel's father that all things are made of chemicals. There are no good chemicals and bad chemicals. There are only good effects and bad effects. Whether they come from the laboratory or the garden, chemicals have no essential nature of goodness or badness. Therefore, whether they are of herbal origin or come from a pill bottle, what is important is what they do and how they do it, not who makes it.

Essiac has many believers. Some contend that the medical profession suppresses it because we are afraid of letting people know that there is a way to get better without the unpleasant options we offer. Do they really believe we want people to suffer? We gain nothing by watching patients endure the difficult options we provide. On the other hand, we only recommend treatments that we know have a reasonable prospect of succeeding. Treatments which are unproved, that put patients at risk by virtue either of their side effects or by postponing urgently needed therapy, are unacceptable to most modern clinicians.

The supporters of such unsubstantiated work fail to recognize the well-known and unexplained incidence of spontaneous remissions (improvements) which occur in many diseases as well as the significant impact of the placebo effect. This latter effect, that is the occurrence of a change in a patient's symptoms or signs due to the use of a neutral or powerless substance, has much to do with the popularity of some herbal preparations. It is a restatement of the important logical trap of post hoc, ergo propter hoc. After the fact, therefore because of the fact. The cock crows, therefore the sun rises. I drink blue green algae every day and I feel better, therefore the blue green algae makes me better, a totally false conclusion with no basis in fact. In the case of consuming blue green algae, a useless substance akin to eating the cuttings from the mowing of your front lawn, this deception is probably harmless except for the impressive and foul smelling gas it produces. In other instances it has been not only harmful, but in some cases fatal.

A few useful illustrations will help to make my point. An important theory regarding the genesis of cancer suggests that compounds called free radicals in the body are causes for many forms of cancer and degenerative illnesses. In the laboratory the effects of free radicals can be neutralized by blocking a chemical reaction which turns chemicals into free radicals. These are called anti-oxidants because they block the oxidation of chemicals and thus prevent damage. Once this was clear, there was a dramatic rush to add anti-oxidants to daily supplements. As I described earlier, the outcome of this process was an unexpected increase in lung cancer in smokers who were taking extra antioxidants, specifically beta-carotene. Suddenly, most of the natural remedy proponents dropped their call for betacarotene. Tryptophan was being pushed for a while by herbalists and holistic clinics for its benefit in helping sleep, reducing the risk of dementia, and lord knows what else. Unfortunately, the Japanese laboratory which prepared the bulk of tryptophan for the American market had a little problem. The substance caused a peculiar inflammatory reaction in the body tissues which caused some people to become quite sick. Hence, no more pushing of tryptophan.

Vitamin B6 (pyridoxine) in small doses is an essential element. In larger doses there is some subjective evidence that it might help to prevent menstrual cramps and in selected patients, reduce heart disease. In pharmacologic doses it can cause damage to the nerves far out from the center of the body, particularly in the hands and feet. Usually this is reversible with stopping the vitamin-but not always. Ma Huang is one of the more recent lethal herbal preparations to have caused disastrous side effects. Touted for its ability to increase energy and stamina, it found wide acceptance in the eager herbal and holistic community. Unfortunately, the primary active agent in Ma Huang is a medication known as ephedrine, a powerful stimulant used in small doses in some prescriptions and in derivatives found in over the counter cold preparations. People who took Ma Huang often felt GREAT!

A 27 year old operator of a surfing and beach sports shop told me about a wonderful supplement he used which gave him more energy. While he was taking it, he found his workouts at the gym went better, and he was able to lift more weight. He stopped it after a month because he thought he should try to do more on his own, thank goodness, and because of the cost. Since he stopped, he noticed he didn't achieve the levels he noted during the month of over-stimulation. I asked for the name of the supplement he was using. We checked out the contents and found that it contained Ma Huang. When I explained to him that this was a highly potent chemical that caused over-stimulation of the cardiovascular and nervous system, he was horrified. Fortunately, he had stopped using the supplement before any damage was done. Many who use this substance have similar effects. They have lots of energy and a substantial subjective feeling of improvement. Sadly, this over-stimulation has led to death in some and medical complication in others.

This is not to deny that some natural herbally derived treatments have great value. Clearly, many herbs and natural substances have important healing power. I am well aware of the tremendously useful herbs and plants used not only by primitive cultures, but even by early American society and still widely accepted in much of Western Europe and the Far East. I also recognize that the utility of many of these preparations is due to the presence of chemical compounds that have been mass-produced by the world pharmaceutical industry in more standardized pills and solutions.

For example, snakeweed, a common flowering substance which grows freely in the southwestern United States, was used for centuries by Native Americans to treat snake bite and other skin problems, as well as fever and many other maladies. I was informed by Paul Torres, a particularly well-informed guide on a recent trip to Arizona, that snake weed is effective because its active ingredient is a salicyclate——aspirin! He pointed out many different species of plants found all around on the trails which had well established effectiveness in treating many ills and complaints. Each is now known to contain compounds which can be purchased at the local pharmacy or supermarket as pain medication, antidiarrheal agents, skin lotions, sedatives and the like.

Aspirin, quinine, digitalis, penicillin, streptomycin, several important blood pressure medicines, zinc, melatonin, saw palmetto among others all have the ability to prolong life or improve its quality for some of us. For others, however, their effects can range from harmless but of no benefit to extremely toxic and sometimes fatal.

What makes many of the items on this list different and the reason why we call them drugs and not potions or tonics is that they have been tested. We understand something about how they work and their potentially dangerous side effects. When we use them, it is in carefully determined amounts that are reasonably standardized. We have some understanding of how they interact with other drugs and with different states of disease.

Aspirin, for example, while valuable for its ability to block inflammation, reduce fever and relieve pain can, when used in children with some viral illnesses, lead to a serious disease called Reye's syndrome which affects the brain and liver. When used to treat pain and inflammation for long periods of time it can lead to kidney damage and bleeding with hemorrhage from the gastrointestinal tract. A memorable aspirin story resulted when one of the greatest professors of medicine, a world-renowned cardiologist, was admitted to a local community hospital here in Boston with a massive gastrointestinal hemorrhage from the small dose of aspirin he was taking to prevent heart attack.

The important distinction between the herbalists and what they like to refer to as traditional western medicine is that, though our treatments may be equally dangerous and perhaps more potent, we have the ability to watch for side effects and know how to treat them. When I start a patient on medicine for her blood pressure, I have specific goals that I can measure with a blood pressure cuff. When the patient returns for a follow-up visit, I know that I must check for symptoms and signs of side effects and to order specific blood tests to determine if problems are developing. I also know that regardless of the risk of side effects, based on the results of studies on hundreds of thousands of patients, they will live a longer and better quality life because we (the patient and I) have controlled the problem.

That's the essential difference- a specific problem, a clear goal, measurable endpoints and an awareness and ability to monitor for risks. Open a package or read an article about some herbal preparation and you will be amazed at what they promise. A bottle of pills containing vitamins and herbs which I recently purchased promised increased strength and endurance, better skin, improved sexual potency, and a greater ability to prevent infections and colds. Who could possibly resist such a promise? There is, however, little scientific evidence to support these claims other than testimonials and indirect inferences from basic research.

The example I get most worked up about presently is echanacea, perhaps one of the most vile smelling and tasting substances I have ever encountered. A few laboratory studies have shown this substance to stimulate aspects of the immune systems. This has been extrapolated to mean that taking echanacea in a liquid or powder form will prevent illness. Whether or not this is true has not been subjected to careful clinical study, nor is there any work of consequence looking into the long-term effects of taking this substance regularly. One bit of promotional material I picked up at a vitamin store mentioned that the American Indians used echinacea as a remedy centuries ago. What they fail to mention is that the Native Americans, while they were indeed in some degree of harmony with nature, also had a substantially shorter life expectancy than the average American today. Although we are far from being in harmony with nature today, that harmony is not likely to be returned to us just by eating vitamins and chanting a daily mantra.

If one allows for the lack of standardization, the uncertainty of dosing, the unknown potential for unpleasant and dangerous side effects, how can a responsible physician recommend substances based on such outlandish claims. Even if one accepts the positive though intellectually dishonest value of the placebo effect, this is a treacherous path to follow. When I give an antibiotic for an infection, I warn the patient of the more common side effects. If anything unusual develops, I can expect to hear from her immediately, whether or not the antibiotic is causing the problem. One patient I recall phoned in an hour after taking a new antibiotic for a severe urinary tract infection. "It's giving me indigestion and gas." A quick flip through my memory led to my response. "But Mrs. Reynolds, you always have indigestion and gas. What's different about it this time?" I knew that it was unlikely for this antibiotic to cause this particular symptom, particularly this quickly. I convinced her to continue with the medication and her complaints diminished over several days.

On the other hand, if I had recommended Goldenseal or liver-wort or Jimson weed and she called with a side effect, I could only refer to the collected wisdom of multiple unstandardized and poorly researched books on herbs or the advice of an herbalist whose knowledge was based on similar texts, word of mouth and personal experience. What am I to say if six months later the patient develops kidney or liver failure, loses her hearing, develops numbness in her hands and feet, finds her hair falling out, develops heart failure or some other unpleasant or catastrophic malady? Is there an herbal manufacturer I can call who has carefully studied thousands of patient responses? Does the National Institute of Health maintain an adverse herb report system? Such protection does not yet exist.

Until we can be certain of the therapeutic value and potential risks of taking large numbers of pills and potions made up of various and sundry natural substances it is wisest to use caution. I advise my patients to be as critical about the supplements as they are about taking any medication or drug. Remember that in addition to many useful medications, a long list of natural substances once thought to be safe are now known to be quite dangerous. A short but memorable list would have to include tobacco, cocaine, mercury, lead, arsenic... and Ma Huang. I am not opposed to the use of natural substances. All I ask for is common sense. Multivitamins yes; Vitamin C yes, in moderation; Vitamin E yes, but no more than 400 units; Aspirin yes, if you can tolerate it; Vitamin B6, no more than 50 mg unless other indications exist; Folic acid yes, but no more than 5 mg; Saw palmetto, try it to see if it works; Ginseng who knows, there is no evidence yet of long term danger; other plants, trees, grasses, powders and potions- let's see some hard scientific data.

In spite of these strong convictions, I must admit that I recently succumbed to the attraction of herbal therapy. During a recent course of my wife's chemotherapy I came down with a simple cold. I felt it coming on about mid morning when I was sitting in the office listening to a patient. That scratchy, dripping feeling in the back of the throat was unmistakable. Like many patients have told me in the past, I just couldn't afford to be sick as my wife's immunity dropped from her treatment.

At Betsy's insistence, I agreed to try echanacea when I went home that evening. I carefully measured out the prescribed number of drops and mixed it with orange juice. This concoction made it barely palatable. Holding my nose to avoid the pungent odor, I swallowed it down in one gulp. I was careful not to breathe in the aroma left over in the glass before I rinsed it down the sink. My wife smiled and I grimaced. Twice a day over the next three days I dutifully repeated the same act with my wife watching. Although I continued to develop a full-blown upper respiratory viral infection with aching and fever, cough and sneezing, sore throat and uncomfortable sinuses, I became aware of a surprising eagerness on my part to take each next dose. Rather than avoid the treatment, I found myself looking forward to taking positive action against this most stubborn foe. I felt good that I was trying to do something to ward off the illness and not just let it happen. I quit after three and half days because the echanacea was obviously not helping.

This experience helped me to better understand the motivation of my patients who try alternative remedies when traditional medicine tells them there is nothing to do. Taking a mysterious mixture of substances that come from nature gives one a sense of action against natural and unnatural forces. It removes a sense of powerlessness and uncertainty. To paraphrase many of my patients, just because science hasn't proved it works doesn't mean it doesn't, right? Well, maybe it does and maybe it doesn't. Much work needs to be and is being done to try to understand more about the nature of action, effects and side effects of some herbal remedies. I await the results of these studies with interest and reserved skepticism.

One final point needs to be made about herbal and vitamin remedies. When I prescribe a drug or therapy to a patient, it is based on my understanding of the problem and the effect of the medication or therapy. I have no financial interest in choosing a particular treatment. On the other hand, in spite of their professed interest in your health, purveyors of vitamin and herbal remedies make a profit on every pill you buy. The testimonials they use from researchers and biochemists are all paid for as part of promotional expenses. Make no mistake about it, the vitamin and health food industry is a very big business. Its major interest is not primarily to make you well but to make a profit.

# *11*

## THE ROAD NOT TAKEN: ALTERNATIVE MEDICINE

Mary Ellen is a 37 year old woman who has come to see me year after year complaining about her aches and pains, her fatigue and her general dissatisfaction with the way she felt. Her diagnosis of choice was usually predicated on what she had read in a magazine or had been told by some less than scrupulous health care provider. Last year it was chronic fatigue syndrome. I agreed with her that she indeed had problems which were present for a long time and therefore chronic, and she certainly was fatigued. Based on the absence of most of the criteria for the disease description I could not, however, confirm the diagnosis of chronic fatigue syndrome. We decided she would pursue some alternative form of treatment since all the standard medicines for her various and sundry complaints appeared to be of little if any benefit. Not only did she feel bad, but she wasn't enjoying life. I suggested meditation, acupuncture, perhaps a prolonged vacation.

When she arrived for her most recent visit, I prepared myself for the usual litany of complaints and her latest self-diagnosis. I had an inkling something had changed when she didn't immediately pull out pages of notes. She appeared more relaxed than I expected and in unusually good spirit as well. Rather than slouching into the chair in my office, shoulders hanging low and face drawn with the expected look of worry, she sat upright and alert. To my surprise, when asked how she was feeling and how the past year had progressed, she responded with a firm and upbeat "Great!" I must admit, I was a little skeptical and was sure she was setting me up to accept her latest imagined malady. I grilled her with my standard series of questions known in medical parlance as the "review of systems." In spite of my persistence, it was clear she truly felt wonderful. She had none of her usual headaches, lack of energy, sleeplessness, irritability, gas or indigestion. Rather than bemoaning her aching joints, she trivialized these and tossed them off with the comment, "What do you expect? This body has to have a few aches and pains."

This was not the Mary Ellen I knew for almost 11 years. What, I asked had happened? From where did she find this new sense of well-being. Proudly, she informed me that she had taken up Tai Chi. In the course of explaining how she learned of this ancient Asian form of movement and exercise, she became quite animated. It was clear she was hooked. By learning to use her body and understand its power, she had found confidence not only in her physical potential, but also in her strength as an individual. Traditional Western Medicine had misled her to think she suffered from illnesses for which we would come up with neatly categorical names. At the same time, my ineptitude in relieving her of these symptoms forced her to seek another way to health. Now she felt in charge and in control. Her attitude to illness and life were completely changed. Her experience is one of many such stories I have encountered over my years in practice which have taught me to believe in the value of what some would call "alternative therapy."

Patients have shown me the therapeutic value of these many different approaches to problems encountered in the daily practice of medicine and in life. It is difficult for some health care providers to accept the impotence of traditional medicine when faced with some difficult and chronic issues. Often we have little to offer or the options for treatment are less than desirable due to side effects and poor responses. Through patients with these types of difficulties, I was exposed to acupuncture, therapeutic massage, chiropractic therapy, yoga, tai chi and other forms of reaffirming mental conditioning as well as movement and exercise practices. I have been awed and humbled by the effectiveness of some of these approaches in helping patients who did not respond or could not tolerate treatments which I prescribed. Accordingly, I have endeavored to seek out practitioners of these arts and skills who I felt were not charlatans and would share my goals of providing relief to the acute symptoms and guidance in long term health maintenance. These practitioners have been willing to work with me, maintaining a connection to scientifically based Western Medicine.

The results have been variable, as expected. Some patients gained great benefit from pursuing these alternative treatments, while others saw little change. This is true of most therapeutic options, regardless of whether they are traditional or alternative. Nothing works for everybody. Sometimes you help and other times not. Unlike traditional medicine, however, these alternative therapies have very little downside risk. Therefore, the failures don't negate the successes as long as the risk of pursuing the treatment is reasonably small. Just as the use of vitamin E and C mentioned in the previous chapter is not of absolute proven benefit, their safety and potential for gain outweighs any potential risk. In this way, the treatments listed above are in most cases safe and without significant risk.

My exposure to alternative medicine began in a rather negative manner when, as a third year medical student rotating through the surgical emergency room at Boston City Hospital, I saw a young Chinese man with what later turned out to be tuberculosis. His back was covered with the red burn rings which I learned were the result of the application of heated glasses or cups to the back- a procedure appropriately known as "cupping". The theory behind this treatment is that the application of heat and the suction created by cooling of the hot glass had the power to draw illness out of the body. This concept of drawing disease out by applying some mechanical external force to the body is a vestige of the dark ages or even some more primitive time. Disease was then seen as the effect of "bad humors" or "bad spirits" on a healthy soul. This seemed to me at the time like a dangerous sort of foolishness, particularly in view of the potentially fatal and highly contagious nature of my patient's illness.

During the next year of medical school and three years of training in a highly academic hospital treating large numbers of patients with diabetes, heart disease, blood disorders and cancer, I saw very little in the way of alternative medicine and developed a rather skeptical attitude to its various manifestations. I learned there were two ways to treat illness- the Harvard way and the wrong way. We were scientifically trained doctors. We found illness, diagnosed and treated and people responded. If they improved, it was because of our careful application of scientific principles. If they didn't get better, it was because they didn't follow the wise advice of scientific medicine, or alternatively, because they got to us too late in their illness for science to do its stuff. We stood by their bedsides and administered drugs which made them feel awful because we knew in the end they would be cured or at least helped. We gave little thought to the effects of food, nutritional supplements, mental attitude or spirituality on the course of their illness. Sure, we knew these factors were important to help people through an illness. We never considered that somehow these non-scientific measures could actually change the course of an illness. Today, most caring practitioners of medicine are open to treatments or life style modification which has some real or imagined capacity to help with little or no downside risk.

One possible exception to this rule of low risk margin with reasonable potential for efficacy is chiropractic treatment. This approach is so controversial in the traditional medical community that it requires a closer look. I believe chiropractic medicine has gained a bad reputation because, like western traditional medicine, there are many bad practitioners. Bad doctors are seen as simply bad doctors. Bad chiropractors are seen as emblematic of an entire profession that is then painted with the same broad brush. Chiropractic medicine is centered on the assumption that much of what ails humans is due to structural misalignments in the skeleton. Careful manipulation of these disturbances is thought to be able to restore comfort and health. To achieve this, chiropractors have developed over the years a panoply of positions, manipulations, massages, twists and pulls which are designed to gradually bring the body back into alignment. Using these techniques, chiropractors are often able to restore comfort to patients in acute and often severe pain. Countless patients unable to gain relief from anti-inflammatory medications, rest, heat and muscle relaxants, the traditional approach, have brought to me stories of immediate relief after one visit to the chiropractor.

I find such stories humbling. These patients come to me with obvious pain, unable to carry on their normal activities, and all I have to offer is medication with side effects, uncomfortable splints and braces, prolonged physical therapy of unproven value and reassurance that with time it will get better. They want immediate relief. As a result, once I am reasonably certain there is no serious underlying medical problem of an urgent or obvious nature, I will often recommend a visit to one of the chiropractors in whom I have developed confidence. Many patients stare in amazement, unable to accept or believe that a very traditional appearing physician could countenance such a referral. Some refuse to embark on this course. Others, however, cautiously proceed with the referral that comes with a warning. If you don't experience prompt improvement within a few visits, return to see me for further evaluation. Though I initially expected limited results, I now frequently receive calls of appreciation for the option to choose this approach. Some will return and go on to additional medical studies and possibly end up on medication or in the hands of a surgeon. Others, however, find a new way to deal with their symptoms and complaints. I have come to accept chiropractic medicine, when practiced thoughtfully and in a cooperative fashion, to be part of the treatment plan I can offer to my patients.

In the same manner, I learned of the value of acupuncture in helping patients suffering from a large and varied number of medical problems. My introduction began when I was accepted to medical school. David, my older brother who was at the time a 60's drop-out from law school living an "alternative life style" in the Haight-Ashbury section of San Francisco sent me a book on Eastern Medicine. I looked with skepticism on the diagrams of meridians and pathways. How could something so illogical, so unscientific apply to my difficult and ponderous studies of modern medical science? I had little belief or interest in such unproven techniques. In the following years I served as a resident in training at a major Harvard teaching hospital. This was followed by the early stages of my career as a new internist (we were not known as primary care practitioners in those days). I had supreme confidence in my ability to diagnose and treat every illness with which I was confronted. I looked down my nose not only at those who were unable to diagnose, but also at patients who had complaints that were undiagnosable, obviously implying that the problem didn't exist.

Then a fortuitous event occurred. A patient, grateful to me for caring for her mother during the several years and last months of her terminal battle with lymphoma, asked me to represent the traditional view on a TV panel she was conducting on acupuncture and alternative therapy. There I was on television, forced to sit with, listen to and watch in action an honest to goodness, real Chinese doctor of acupuncture. She was not only appreciative of the position of western medicine, but also suggested that I should view acupuncture as an adjunct or cooperative aspect of care. Rather than seeing it as an alternative form of therapy, she encouraged me to seek out ways to use this ancient form of treatment alongside my standard approach.

With this new option, I began to refer patients to her, along with several other acupuncturists I sought in the community. To my surprise, the results for some patients were dramatic. People were able to cope better with illnesses as diverse as chronic back pain, migraine, cancer pain and asthma. For a few sufferers, their symptoms vanished, while for others there was a clear change in attitude. No longer a helpless victim, they gained a sense of control. They had a tool with which to respond to their pain that did not require the administration of medication nor did it place them in the role of passive sufferer. Going to the acupuncturist was an active form of self-help. I found that acupuncture was a useful adjunct in the care of patients with chronic and acute problems. While it did not appear to be the magic cure many had presented to me, it was quite clear that I needed to include acupuncture as an alternative form of therapy.

My impression of Yoga began in much the same way. The image I carried derived largely from childhood Saturday morning cartoons of turban-wearing characters twisted into pretzel-like positions. Like many men, I have never been able to sit cross-legged in what is known as the lotus position. The entire process of achieving inner peace through such painful self-manipulation seemed ludicrous. Attempts to fold foot under opposite thigh in an effort to mimic the pose resulted in either intolerable hip pain or a humiliating fall to the side.

In spite of this disbelief, patients repeatedly told me of the stimulation and sense of relaxation and near euphoria they achieved by performing their daily exercises. My interest was particularly peaked by the wife of one of our senior radiologists. She always appeared to possess the essence of calm and composure. Whether it was her natural disposition or the benefits of Yoga, listening to her made me more receptive to the notion that there must be some value to this stuff. About the same time, some interesting research from Yale University demonstrated that patients who practiced Yoga and meditation prior to major surgical procedures had easier recoveries, with less need for pain medication and a faster return to normal activity.

With this in mind, I encouraged my wife when a close friend suggested she try yoga and meditation to help her through the distress of her illness and chemotherapy. Although previously she might have rejected such an option, she pursued the sessions, and now views this as an essential part of her treatment. Her appointments are kept as carefully as those with her oncologist. On a recent trip she even induced me to give it another try after she told the instructor of my fearful intimidation by the need to achieve the lotus position. I was assured that the practice of yoga did not require immediate total relaxation. Like most things in life, with a little practice and conditioning I would be able to achieve the proper effect with or without the lotus. To my surprise, I enjoyed the hour-long session. While I didn't take all of the running monologue of our instructor too seriously ("This will stimulate your thyroid and this will stimulate your spleen and immune system."), I did indeed feel paradoxically both relaxed and energized. Now I routinely recommend yoga and meditation to patients faced with a myriad of life's stresses. Whether dealing with an impending surgical problem, coping with cancer and chemotherapy, or simply facing the daily task of addressing life's responsibilities, yoga and meditation appear to help people regain a sense of control.

Just as acupuncture and Tai Chi provide physical relief, and yoga and meditation stimulate a physical sense of well being, they also appear to touch a more spiritual need to separate from the invasive aspects of modern life and, more specifically, modern medicine. At some level, there is an effort in these activities which strives to reach towards some greater force, a centering power. They take on an almost religious intensity. I found this same power during the year after my father's death when I fulfilled my responsibility as a son to attend daily prayer services where, in addition to chanting the traditional liturgy of the service, I would stand with others in mourning to chant the Kaddish. It was necessary to waken even earlier than my usual 4:30 am start in order to finish rounds at the hospital and get to the chapel by the 6:30 beginning of schachris, the morning service. For the first few weeks I often found myself weeping and struggling to get through the chanting without the welling up of emotion which follows such a loss. I found myself recalling standing with my father as he performed the same duty after his parents' deaths. I remembered how hard it was for him at the beginning as well. Yet, as the weeks went on, I recognized a sense of strength and continuity which carried me through the daily acts of putting on my tefillin and tallit, reading psalms with the early arrivals if I managed to get to shul early enough, reading the prayers and reciting the Kaddish. I understood better the benefit of the gentle swaying back and forth during prayer that I watched in my father and grandfathers four decades earlier.

Clearly, religious practices and beliefs provide a great source of strength and reassurance to those who are suffering. It also serves as a source of strength and sustenance to the physically and mentally healthy—sort of a spiritual health maintenance organization. Often, in our work as physicians and scientists we forget the healing value of belief. We tend to see our roles as professionals and technicians with understanding and access to a vast network of information. Like shamans of ancient times, we cloak ourselves in a mantle of power that protects us from the suffering and confusion we witness and treat.

I was reminded of this by a young man whom our congregation was interviewing for the position of chief Rabbi. He chose as his drash or point of discussion the holy nature of the physician's visit to a sick patient. Using religious text, he presented the image of a physician sitting at the bedside of the patient who is surrounded by the holiness of God. Therefore, he argued, visiting and tending to a sick patient was to stand before the presence of the Almighty. The power of this argument changed forever the way I viewed my interaction with patients. More important, it strengthened my already firm belief that skilled pastoral visits by clergy often are more useful to patients than all our intensive medical efforts.

The common threads in all these approaches to healing is a sense of control, of participating in the healing process, of being a part of something greater than individual suffering or discomfort. Whether by choosing an alternative treatment regimen or the addition of spiritual or metaphysical healing powers, it is clear that most patients need to feel that they have some input into the course of their treatment. Whenever possible, they want a sense of contributing to their health or recovery rather than passively enduring life, illness and treatment.

While many patients need to see their physician as wise and judicious, some of these and others want to know that their immediate and long-term health can be positively affected by their own actions. It is clearly possible to meld these approaches within the scope of traditional western medicine in an attempt to give patients the best of both worlds. I ask practitioners of alternative therapies to work with me. This does not require the active pursuit of an alternative life style nor the exclusive attention of a so-called "holisitic" practitioner. It does, however, require that the physician and patient function as partners in both sickness and wellness. Ultimately this means that patients must accept not only a burden of responsibility for their own well being, but also a sense of being part of something larger than themselves. This acceptance leads to greater feeling of control and lack of dependence on the medical community. At the same time, it represents a choice to be an active participant in health and wellness.

# *12*

## WAITING FOR THE OTHER SHOE TO DROP: THE FEAR OF AGING

**M**ax Cooper, a dear family friend, confided in me at dinner recently that at 81, in spite of his vigorous good health, he felt like the character in an old story he had heard. He told me of the fellow who came home late one night and quickly disrobed. Without thinking, he dropped his first shoe heavily on the floor, which of course woke his neighbor one floor below. Not wanting to disturb others further, he more carefully and gently placed his other shoe down so as not to create any excessive noise. An hour later, his neighbor called from downstairs to complain that he was unable to sleep because he had been waiting for the other shoe to drop so he could again enjoy his rest. Max was only half serious in telling the story because he remains one of the most vigorous and active senior citizens I know, and in truth, has very little time to worry about his own mortality. But he admitted subsequently to feeling disturbed as he watched his friends and acquaintances of equal years dropping off around him. He worries about the prospects for infirmity, dependence and pain.

These fears and concerns are a common theme in my visits with the elderly. While most recognize that life is finite and all will come to an end at some point, it is the dangers and insecurities of disability and aging which they fear the most. Like the line from the musical "Showboat", they are mostly "tired o' livin, but scared o' dyin." And why should they not fear the normal changes that occur? Television depicts the elderly as being vibrant and alert, mentally sharp and certainly without the difficulties of leaky bladders, failing memory, insomnia, disabling pain, abandonment by families, loneliness and dependency in nursing homes. Although manufacturers of products to assist with these problems abound, their advertisements usually consist of an elderly individual or couple living a joyous life working, traveling, fishing or visiting with the grandchildren through the use of their nutritional supplement, diaper, denture adhesive, arthritis medication or laxative.

The elderly know that these images, though appealing, are far from the lives they experience. The most common phrase I hear from my older patients is "It's no good to be old." In fact, I hear it so often, at one point I wondered if the phrase had been printed on some senior citizen bathroom wall where they could all pick it up to repeat just to me. I know from colleagues, however, that this is a common refrain. After reviewing the usual long list of medications and reciting a multitude of complaints, the elderly patient will often sigh, "Who called these the golden years?"

While the pace of illness and catastrophic events increases as we age, much of the difficulty confronting the elderly is not a sign of impending doom. Rather, these common and annoying difficulties represent part of a natural aging process. Efforts to "fix" them often create more problems than they help. These include the issues of memory loss, sleep disturbances, fatigue, joint pains and loss of appetite. Clearly these can all be signs of serious underlying disease in need of medical attention. It is important to have a good relationship with a general medical doctor (an internist or family practitioner) who can investigate the problems and determine if they represent issues of greater concern. Once this has been ruled out, however, it is important to learn to recognize the nature of the problems and deal with them, rather than to allow a difficulty to become a major focus and hence, a force which destroys quality of life.

Probably the most common complaint in this category is loss of memory. We have become so terrified of the possibility of Alzheimer's disease that any loss of memory is seen as the beginning of the end. People come in at all ages fearful because they were unable to remember the name of an old friend they had not seen in 5 years or because they forgot a grandchild's birthday. Perhaps they forgot to put the soup back in the refrigerator the night before or missed an appointment because they just didn't remember. Terrified, they present, sometimes in tears, certain that Alzheimer's disease is imminent and that it is only a matter of a short time before they will be vegetating in a nursing home bed, alone and forgotten.

By making this diagnosis more visible, the medical profession has both improved our ability to diagnose the problem, but has also created a new bogey-man for the elderly to fear. In the pre-Alzheimer days, the elderly could look at this process and call it "hardening of the arteries" or just "getting a little soft" in old age. Now, with a diagnosis and clear picture as to the course, the fear has a name and a face. Most elderly patients know someone who has suffered this diagnosis and watched the slow and unpleasant deterioration of connection to the real world. They have seen these individuals lose their personality and become progressively dependent and incompetent, ultimately placed in an extended care facility so that low paid staff can attempt to keep them clean and fed while the professionals attempt to maintain the highest level of function possible for each patient. Slowly, they fade as family and friends wait for the inevitable. Given this scenario, it is understandable why a patient would be terrified at the slightest sign of loss of memory.

The good news is that most people don't get Alzheimer's disease and most people lose some memory as time goes by. It is such a common process that it has become one of the greatest sources of health related jokes. Clearly, one of the ways we as a culture deal with issues about which we have the greatest fear is to make them objects of humor. Our laughter weakens the evil we face while at the same time it enables us to confront our fear. The truth is, however, that we all lose some memory. Forgetting names, phone numbers, appointments, glasses, birthdays, keys, scientific formulas, recipes, words to songs-these are all normal occurrences as individual events. Medical concern arises if the memory loss is more complex. For example, while any one or two of the above list is no reason for concern, a collection of them would be more worrisome. That is to say it is a real matter for concern if you forget your neighbor's name one day and a week later miss an important appointment, and then find yourself unable to put together your old recipe for brownies. This does not mean, however, that you have Alzheimer's disease. There are many causes for memory loss, often of a reversible nature.

Some are as common as stress reactions, underactive thyroid function and simple vitamin deficiency states, while others may involve more complex issues such as correctable changes in brain pressure or treatable depression. What it does mean is that you need to see your doctor who will examine you and perform some simple tests looking for one of the many reversible causes of memory loss. Once this has been performed and all the more serious causes are ruled out, assuming the memory loss is of the more characteristic "normal" type, it is time to stop worrying about this and get on with life.

Sleep disturbances are the second largest group of complaints presented by the elderly. The causes are often so simple and so obvious that patients find them hard to accept. While we all require a certain amount of sleep to get through the day, that amount is not dependent on some magical formula we are given by our mothers when we are young. Rather, a multitude of factors affect the duration of necessary sleep. These include the amount of activity experienced in the course of the day, medications taken, consumption of caffeine, alcohol and tobacco, emotional stresses, ambient noise and light factors, recent time zone changes. Everybody knows that if you spend the day working outside with a shovel digging a ditch, carrying snow or moving dirt, you will sleep much better that night than if you spend the day reading this book. Of course, you should still read this book and pursue other activities that are not overly physical. The point is that older people are, in general, less physically active. Therefore, they use less energy and require less sleep. When questioned about their state of energy in the morning, those who seem to require less sleep are unaware of any sense of unusual fatigue. They are just not happy about being up at 4:30 in the morning when there isn't much to do and are unable to go back to sleep.

There are options to deal with this problem. While it can be an unpleasant prospect for the first one to two weeks, weaning oneself off caffeine can go a long way to restoring a normal sleep cycle. Caffeine, while energizing and stimulating, is a drug which can have lasting effects. As we get older, our ability to limit the effects of all drugs and chemicals is weakened. This permits the effects of drugs, in this place caffeine, to linger much longer and with greater intensity than when we were younger. If you're going to continue some caffeine, don't compound the effects by having any late in the day. You should avoid caffeine after noon. Remember also that caffeine is present in cola beverages, tea and chocolates. Eliminating liquids in general after 7 PM at night, except during heat waves, will reduce the need to waken at night to empty the bladder. Increasing exercise on a daily basis will not only help to restore your sleep-wakefulness pattern, but also restore normal levels of brain chemicals that help to facilitate a healthy sleep pattern.

It is also important to review your medications with your doctor to be certain that nothing needs to be changed because of possible side effects. Don't assume that the doctor is always aware of this possibility. There are plenty of times when patients have brought this to my attention when I had not considered it as part of the problem, even when the drug manufacturers did not mention sleeplessness as a potential side effect. Most important, as with all non-serious medical issues, don't sit and fret about your inability to sleep the mandatory 8 hours a night. The more you worry about it, the less you'll sleep.

Some will say "I've tried all that and I still can't sleep. I lie awake at night and never close my eyes." In the absence of a significant problem with thyroid function or a major psychiatric disorder, nobody will stay awake forever. Sooner or later, the body will fall asleep out of simple exhaustion. Yet people contend that they can't bear another night without sleep, and so we prescribe sleeping pills. The sedative market has always been an enormous source of revenue to the pharmaceutical industry representing billions of dollars in sales. Drug manufacturers have gone so far as to advertise their brands to the public through the standard broadcast and paper media in an effort to build demand for their particular drug.

While there is little doubt these medicines work, their effectiveness comes at a cost. Most are derived from a family of drugs known as benzodiazepines. These drugs can cause depression, memory loss and difficulty with motor skills. Often, contrary to the drug companies' denials, they can cause disturbances in daytime alertness, the so-called "hang-over" effect. Typically they lose their effectiveness over time and have a uniform potential to cause dependency and addiction. Although there are certainly some patients who can use these medicines carefully and infrequently with safety, in general it is better to deal with sleeplessness as described above rather than opting for the medical approach. And if you can't sleep, then read a book, or even better, write one. However you deal with sleeplessness, don't worry about it. You will eventually fall asleep.

The third most common complaint of the elderly is sore joints. Another internist I know calls this the "Falling Hand Syndrome." As part of the routine evaluation, an internist will ask if there is any joint pain, at which point an elderly patient is likely to reply either "You know, the usual. Nothing important." or alternatively, slowly moving the hands to indicate the location of the discomfort, "My neck and my back, my shoulders, and mostly my thumb. Also my hips when I get up and my knees have been worse lately. And the feet- Oh the feet are so sore." Now it is important to recognize that all these areas probably do hurt. Also, one can assume that all the common causes of joint pain have been eliminated by the time I ask this question of a regular patient.

So the issue then becomes how to allow this patient to accept a chronic problem while still providing some modicum of relief. The first step is to help the patient understand that deterioration of the joints is a natural phenomenon. Our joints are made of living material that responds to the normal stresses of weight bearing and movement. Like shock absorbers on cars and upholstery on furniture, the more use they get, the more wear that occurs on the bearing surfaces. The nice cushy surface of each joint formed by the smooth pliable cartilage that the Original Designer created takes the brunt of the force and over time, gradually deteriorates and wears away. This exposes the bony underlying surface to wear and tear and which leads to pain. It happens to everybody, and most particularly those who have the good fortune of living long enough. At the same time, the muscles and ligaments that hold it all together also loosen with age. Pain in the joints and altered movement created by the response to that pain puts extra loads on these structures and causes spasm and pain. There is no way to avoid some degree of this problem as time goes on. Gravity is unavoidable and the consequences are part of the human condition.

This is not to say that nothing can be done to reduce the severity and ameliorate the development of arthritic pain. Sometimes the pain can be severe and incapacitating. Having injured my neck in wrestling in high school, I know well the effects of persistent, nagging, gnawing discomfort for days on end. It can wear you down and even make you feel a little depressed and irritable. At 35, 40, 45 and even 50, it can be an annoyance, but at least you know you have many days ahead that will be pain-free. When you're 75 and over, you don't have the patience for days of pain when you're wondering how many days you have left in total. The elderly are appropriately impatient with pain. The options for treatment that we can offer can be helpful.

First and most important is the recognition that the problem is chronic and will not go away completely. Therefore, treatment is aimed at maintaining flexibility and providing temporary relief from discomfort. Most studies now indicate that remaining physically active, no matter how crippled or incapacitated an individual may be, helps to strengthen bones and improve the suppleness of joints and resistance to injury. That is to say, the more active you remain in your advancing years, the more resistant you will be to progression of the degenerative process. Even in nursing home bound patients, it is quite clear that daily physical activity of some sort reduces the risk of falls and improves overall bodily function. The more sedentary you become, the more prone you will be to injury and disability. The key concept is - use it or lose it.

Treating chronic pain of arthritis in the elderly is more complicated than the purveyors of "arthritis strength" medication would have us believe. Traditional arthritis medications, the group known as non-steroidal anti-inflammatory drugs (NSAIDs), may help to reduce pain but carry significant risks in the elderly which are greater than in young people. This is primarily due to the changes that occur in the body as it ages. For example, they alter the flow of blood in the kidneys in a way that can damage kidney function. This can be of minimal significance in a young healthy person, but can pose a major risk in older patients whose kidney blood supply is already compromised by the effects of aging on small blood vessels. NSAIDs can irritate the wall of the stomach and cause bleeding. This does not happen often, but in older patients where the stomach empties more slowly, the risk of bleeding becomes greater. Older people are more likely to be on multiple other medications that can have bad interactions and lead to greater problems. Most important, for the degenerative and non-inflammatory pain of wear and tear arthritis, it is apparent that plain old tylenol (acetominophen) works as well for the pain. Even tylenol is not without risk when taken for long periods at high doses. At a low dosage level started at advanced age and used sporadically, it is probably safe.

Some new and alternative approaches to pain in the elderly have proven helpful. These include modalities as complex as injections of the powerful drug cortisone into the areas of pain under the supervision of a trained anesthesiologist or orthopedic surgeon. Other equally intriguing but very opposite options involve the use of chiropractic manipulation, acupuncture, biofeedback and some herbal forms of treatment. Although there are no good controlled trials with these forms of treatment, the risk is low and I have seen patients gain tremendous benefit in selected cases. Many patients look at me in astonishment when I suggest that we try acupuncture for their unremitting back pain. In the hands of a skilled and sensitive practitioner of this form of treatment, I have seen good results. The only real down side is that very few insurance companies will pay for the treatments, but that's an issue for another time.

Regardless of which approach is used, the key to remember is that some soreness and "creakiness" is natural. If you develop new pain in your joints or your back that won't go away or gets progressively worse over time, you should consult your primary care physician. If no cause is apparent and you're confident that you have been thoroughly evaluated, don't worry about those aching bones. In the words of an elderly and spry gentleman who sees me only once a year, if he woke up in the morning and nothing hurt, it would mean he was dead.

In spite of this depressing picture, there is always a group who either has no complaints or, more typically, finishes the review of problems with a twinkle in their eye or a wonderful story. I know in advance who this will be because their visit often begins with an inquiry as to my health and my family. Their world extends beyond their own discomfort and mortality. Although this may represent a need to deflect interest and discussion about the patient's problems, it also demonstrates an interest and awareness that extends beyond the tip of their nose. So many of my patients see the world of illness, aging and infirmity only as it relates to them. Their experience is limited to some imaginary space that surrounds them and their activities. As a result it is hard for them to view the aging process as part of a natural cycle and accept their lot in life for the inevitable process it represents. This prevents them from gaining joy from the daily occurrences and major events that mark all our lives. If all you see is sadness in the passing of life's energy, how can you appreciate the beauty of a sunset, the song of a bird, the smell of a rose, the laugh of a child, a grandchild's graduation or marriage.

I am inspired constantly by my patients who are able to look beyond their personal suffering and misfortune, which most of us are likely to experience, and still find a reason to waken each day with a smile. Though many patients have shown me this inner strength, one particular patient stands out. I use her real name because I know she served as an inspiration to her family as well. Bessie Andrews was an elderly woman who lived alone in Boston and suffered from severe and debilitating arthritis. Her joints had been worn over the years by both an active life and the ravages of inflammatory rheumatoid disease. She suffered not only the effects of the disease, but also complications from the many medications she received over the years to keep the inflammatory process at bay.

In spite of this, she always came to see me with a smile and a story. She saved her complaints until she reached a point where life was unbearable. Although she lived alone, she had an attentive family who lived in a distant part of the country. I heard from her daughters often, particularly as she began to fail in strength and lose weight. Our ability to investigate her problems was limited by her frailty and her tendency to minimize her difficulties. Finally, when it became impossible for her to live alone, her daughter had her move to her home in another state. We said a sincere good by, with comments about her returning to see me soon, knowing full well she would not return.

Shortly after arriving at her daughter's home, her condition deteriorated rapidly and she soon died of a malignancy that is occasionally associated with her chronic illness. Little could have been done to prevent or change this course. Thankfully, her daughter called me to give me the news. I told her how much I would miss her mother and the air of joy she carried around her. Bessie knew the end was not far away, in spite of my unsuccessful efforts to the contrary. Yet she kept her life whole by remaining connected with the world, finding joy in even the brief moments she was able to experience, and always understanding her place in the natural order of life. In the words of Rachel Goldberg, an 88 year old woman whom I have had the pleasure of seeing for a number of years, "I can accept a lot if I can get up in the morning and see the sun. Then I know I'm still alive."

# *13*

## THERE MUST BE A PONY SOMEWHERE: LOSING THE FEAR OF CANCER

E va, a 43 year old Russian born computer programmer comes in to see me several times a year. She is attractive, well dressed and poised. On most visits we briefly discuss her husband and daughter who are generally healthy and well adjusted and her work which she clearly enjoys. Within a short ten years after arriving in the United States she and her family have rapidly assimilated and achieved some degree of professional and financial success. Her daughter is flourishing in the public schools and the family lives in a comfortable neighborhood in one of Boston's better suburbs. It was almost as if everything for them was too good.

On her most recent visit I asked the usual detailed questions with which I always begin my evaluation, and she denied any problems in those areas. I then asked her how she was managing with the abdominal pain she has repeatedly complained of in the past. As expected, she reported that the four year old pain is still present. We review various aspects of the problem. It is clear the character and quality of the pain is essentially unchanged. I remind her that we have looked this over repeatedly, including extensive and comprehensive laboratory and gastrointestinal studies, CAT scans, kidney x-rays, evaluation by gastroenterologists, surgeons and gynecologists and have been unable to find any medical disease. I have attempted on many occasions to discuss the relationship of Eva's symptoms to her emotional fears, but she repeatedly resists this approach. Once again, she raises the question as to whether there could be some lurking cancer we have overlooked.

I point out that the pain has remained unchanged for four years. It is not disabling nor is it so severe as to interrupt work, sleep, the ability to socialize or pursue activities that give pleasure. In truth, we have looked in every way imaginable and found no cancer. I try my best to reassure her that she is free of cancer, but I can tell by her demeanor that she is not completely at ease.

Just as with all the illnesses in the previous chapters, many in our culture require this same sense of certainty that they are free of the diagnosis or cancer. It is not enough for them to hear me say all the tests are normal. They respond "How can you be sure?" Often patients will come in requesting a "total body scan". They need some concrete reassurance that they are clear, something which I'm sure would appeal to all of us. The truth is, I can only be sure within a margin of accuracy. The tests are rarely 100 % reliable. X-rays, scans, ultrasounds, MRI's and other high technology equipment all have a less than perfect ability to avoid missing diagnoses. Even biopsies and careful microscopic examination can be subject to error.

I recall a patient with a lung problem which one radiologist read as unequivocal lung cancer, but on biopsy was said to be benign. The patient and his family quite appropriately never forgave me for presenting the likely diagnosis before the specimen was reviewed by a pathologist. Even two years later when he died from the lung cancer that turned out to be there anyway, they sustained their anger. Errors can occur because of location used for tissue sampling. It can also occur if the proper stain doesn't take well to the tissue or if the pathologist happens to miss that one small area of tumor. A wise physician, meaning one who has made the mistake at least once, knows the danger of false reassurance. Yet patients continue to come in looking for a professional pronouncement that they are clean.

This is a story repeated often in medical practices across the country. Many people live in constant fear of developing or already harboring some form of cancer which, if left undiagnosed and untreated, will lead to some horribly painful calamitous end to life. We in the profession have been more than happy to respond to this fear and need for certainty, however false. We unconsciously feed our egos and our wallets by facilitating this process. A sense of foreboding and dread permeates messages sent out to the community by the medical profession, the media and the health care industry.

Who could be blamed for fearing the worst when those who should be reassuring are instead throwing up red flags of warning? Physicians and medical groups try to promote their expertise with newsletters about the latest and hottest screening tests. Commercial and academic clinics for treating cancer are constantly competing in the marketplace using attractive television and newspaper advertisements. The media gets us on two fronts both with health focused items in print and audiovisual offerings as well as heartbreaking movies, books and television stories about the tragedy of cancer. This latter is so common that my wife and I have to screen books and movies in advance to be sure they are not a reheated version of Love Story or Terms of Endearment with a dying spouse, parent or child ravaged by cancer. Even if you didn't want to think about cancer, it is in the air everywhere.

I can certainly understand this fear. My life and that of my family has repeatedly confronted the diagnosis of cancer. I vividly recall being told over the phone by a colleague that the mole I had insisted be removed (after three of the most prominent dermatologists in Boston told me it was nothing) was in fact a melanoma, a potentially aggressive cancer of the skin. It had penetrated deeply into layers that put me at risk for spread. I had to go back into the hospital for more extensive surgery and wait patiently to find out the test results. I subjected myself to regular visits to a melanoma clinic for a couple of years, but finally bailed out since the stress and anxiety these visits created in my family life became unacceptable. Like most people who find out they have cancer, this could not have come at a worse time. My wife was pregnant with our third child. We were just moving into a new house and I had left a group of physicians to start my own practice only the week before. Now, more than 19 years later, I still wonder on occasion if the unusual headache or strange symptom we all feel from time to time may be due to the well known late recurrence of this cancer. More important, I learned about the fear patients carry of missed diagnoses even by the best of physicians. Had I not insisted on the removal of this mole, I would not be sitting writing this book today. Though I rarely worry about the diagnosis of melanoma any more, I know this experience affects my view of patients' complaints, my role as a physician and my attitude to the world in which I live.

During that period our family faced cancer in a three year old niece who died a horribly painful and disabling end from a malignant tumor of the spinal canal. Shortly afterwards, a four year old niece developed leukemia and underwent a daring bone marrow transplant from which she has since fully recovered. Earlier in the book I mentioned the development of lymphoma in my father which dragged on for seven years. Late in my dad's illness, my father-in-law developed an aggressive form of lung cancer from which he has since passed away. I watched both of them as I sat at their bedsides at the very end waiting for the last breath of their living and their suffering. Within a year of this last diagnosis, my wife developed lymphoma and underwent surgery and chemotherapy which is ongoing. We would joke half-heartedly that we were one of the few families in Boston with an oncologist for a family doctor as the three of them, my wife, father and father-in-law would often be found at the oncology clinic together.

All of this occurred on top of my large practice following many patients with similar and sometimes worse diagnoses. Like many of my patients, I sat with my wife through sleepless nights as we anxiously awaited reports from the radiologist on her latest CAT scan. I know what it is like to wait for the phone call on the pathology report, and I know what it is like to have a diagnosis missed or made in error, as well as the feeling a physician experiences when we overlook or miss a diagnosis.

I painfully recall the moment when, sitting in the lounge at my hospital, I received the call from my colleague that he had found a large and extensive tumor in my wife's abdomen. This only two months after one of Boston's greatest specialists suggested that she suffered from chronic fatigue syndrome. It is hard to describe the overwhelming emotion that arises at such a time. Just thinking about it now brings back the lump in the back of the throat and the swelling up of tears familiar to all who have faced this experience in a loved one. I have watched the disruptive impact of this diagnosis on my children. Hardly anybody is free from knowing some close friend or relative who has fallen victim. Because our society is clustered so closely in dense population centers and given the immediacy of modern telecommunication, word of a new diagnosis of cancer spreads rapidly through the community. It would be hard not to perceive all this as a dramatic increase in cancer.

And yet, with only a few exceptions, the incidence of cancer per population has remained unchanged or even diminished. At the same time, the rate of cure has substantially improved. Even in many of those cancers where an increase in new cases diagnosed has been documented, some may be due to our increased ability to find cancers earlier, such as in breast, prostate and colon cancer. In association with this increase in incidence of these tumors has been a decrease in the death rate and an increase in the cure rate. That is to say, we are finding more but in many cases people are dying less. This suggests that some of the increase may be due to statistical factors such as simply diagnosing these tumors so early that we may be finding some which might never become problems at all.

In prostate cancer, for example, there are few physicians who would avoid performing a digital rectal examination and a prostate specific antigen blood test (PSA) annually on every Afro-American male over 40 and every white male over 50 in an effort to find prostate cancer early and then treat. We have been strongly encouraged to do so by the American Cancer society and the National Cancer Institute. The treatment choices now include observation, surgery, radiation, surgery with radiation, radiation with hormonal therapy followed by surgery, radiation pellet implantation and others. The issue becomes clouded when one notes that there is little hard evidence suggesting that picking up very early prostate cancers using this technique prolongs life or improves survival. Given the intense anxiety created by testing, the complications of biopsy and treatment, would the majority of men be better off if we just left their prostates alone? Since the incidence is going up and the cure rate is going up as well, does this mean that more prostate cancer is suddenly appearing? Are we simply diagnosing it so early that it would have resolved on its own, simply regressed spontaneously, or grown so slowly as to never be a significant problem?

It will be many years before we know the correct answer to the question. Very likely we will find a select group who do benefit. The key is to know how to identify that group, perhaps through genetic mapping techniques. In the meantime, tens of thousands of American men are having microscopic tumors found in their prostate glands which are either surgically removed or irradiated. The end result is that men now walk around as obsessively frightened of prostate cancer and its consequences as women have been with breast cancer.

I don't suggest for a moment that patients should drop their vigilance for cancer. There is much we can do to watch for early signs and even prevent its development. Any reasonable physician would recommend regular mammography and breast exams, pap smears, skin exams, oral exams, stool blood exams and periodic sigmoidoscopy, along with the many other important aspects of annual contact with your doctor. In addition, people must be alert to a number of important signs. These include unusual bleeding, sudden and unexplained change in appetite or weight loss that lasts more than a few weeks, significant change in appearance of a skin lesion or rash which lasts more than 3 or 4 weeks, prolonged and unexplained cough, pain which comes with no provocation and doesn't resolve after many weeks or gets progressively worse over a shorter period of time, unexplained and prolonged change in a normal bodily function such as breathing, swallowing, urination, bowel function, sexual function, problems with balance, coordination and use of the extremities, or prolonged and unexplained weakness and fatigue.

Problems in these areas which come on without provocation and persist without explanation require attention. Call your doctor if you have one. Don't call a specialist, clinic, emergency room, hospital information line or the American Cancer Society. Don't go surfing the web. Hopefully you have somebody who knows you and your history and can either reassure you or begin the necessary investigation. If you feel your concern hasn't been taken seriously, say so. If you're still not satisfied, get another evaluation. Once that has been completed and hopefully the results are good, don't go on worrying about the possible diagnosis or the symptoms. Let it go and move on with your life.

So often, coming into the medical process leads to a never-ending array of medical investigations. The self-focus and the concern of others fostered by potential medical difficulties often feeds our need for attention and importance in a very impersonal world. It can be a refuge from the stress of the work environment or may diffuse some of the tension of a dysfunctional family. For the elderly it is often a place to pass time and be certain of care. Remember that wonderful feeling of warmth and security when you stayed home sick from school? When we are adults, a desire for that same warmth and security can lead to frequent medical visits, more tests, more concerned family members, anxious co-workers and friends and neighbors. Everybody gets worked up, and it often leads no where.

In contrast to this obsessive fear of the diagnosis of cancer is the person who deals with his fear by denying the possibility this could ever happen to him. Janet was a perfect example. At age 48 she had avoided medical care for many years, probably since the birth of her only son who was now 17 years old. She came from a very traditional family of Mediterranean origin, and believed that her maternal responsibilities did not include worrying or complaining of her own health. She came in with her husband Tony, ostensibly for a severe respiratory illness. They both appeared remarkably anxious considering the nature of the complaint, so I assumed there was more here than met the eye. My suspicions were confirmed when the husband took me aside while his wife was putting on a gown in the examination room.

"Doc, you got to check her out. I think she has something bad on her chest that she won't show me or anybody else."

I reassured him and proceeded to the next room where I performed my usual exam for a respiratory illness. During the course of this I managed to slip the gown down enough to see an enormous and far advanced tumor of the breast growing through the skin. Rather than confront her in this defenseless and awkward position of near nakedness, I waited until we returned to my office and then presented the facts in a straightforward and non judgemental manner.

"You have a cold which should clear up on its own in a short period of time. Continue to use the same over the counter medicines you have at home. There's another problem which I'm afraid is more serious. The growth which I noticed on your chest needs some attention." She initially looked at me with a blank expression. Then she began to softly cry and then began sobbing. It was as if the flood gates were suddenly allowed to open.

"I didn't know what to do. At first, I thought it was nothing. I mean, I just never worried about my health and never thought anything could happen to me. I thought maybe it would just go away. I didn't want to worry my husband. He had so much on his mind with his job, and my son was just going off to college. I couldn't upset him either at such an important time. So I just kept it to myself. Then it got bigger and I knew something was wrong. I knew it was cancer and I knew what that meant. I saw what happened to my friend once they told her she had breast cancer. It was horrible. She lost her hair and she was so sick. I couldn't put myself and my family through that. Now you'll want to do the same to me." She continued to cry and shake with each sob.

We paused for a moment as I allowed her to collect herself. After she had calmed a little, I asked, "And how is your friend now, the one with the breast cancer?"

"Well she looks fine. But I'm sure what she went through was just horrible."

"But she's fine now. Is that what you're saying?"

"I guess so. She looks pretty normal. Her hair has mostly grown back and I see her all over town at the market and whatever."

"I see. So she was diagnosed with breast cancer, had a lump removed and presumably had extra treatment with chemotherapy, what we call adjuvant or added on therapy, and now she looks and acts pretty normal. This probably means she had a good result from her treatment. With a little luck and good medical care, she may live a full and normal life. Don't you think you're entitled to the same chance to live a full and normal life?"

"I guess so." Her response was less than convincing. We talked a bit about her need to protect her family and her feelings of guilt and shame for getting sick. We discussed her need to understand that she was not the cause of her illness and was not being punished for some wrong done at another time. It took a few phone conversations and another visit. Finally she agreed to go on to the oncologist I recommended for further evaluation and treatment.

When I ask people to not worry about cancer, I don't mean to hide from the diagnosis. Just as Janet got herself in a serious predicament by her avoidance and denial, so she could have wasted part of her life worrying for years about getting breast cancer when there was little she could do to prevent it. That, in essence is my whole point about cancer and worry. You can spend your life worrying about getting it or you can pretend that it never will happen. The truth is, if you're going to get cancer, given the current state of medical knowledge, you will get it whether you worry or not. Since it's out of your control, why bother spending your energy and your life worrying?

Worry is such a destructive force. No useful purpose can be served with energy frittered away to that end. Certainly, take all the necessary precautions we know are effective. Be alert to the warning signs mentioned earlier in this chapter. Get regular checkups each year and be sure to have screening tests such as mammograms, sigmoidoscopies, colonoscopies and PAP smears on a regular basis. If you are so inclined, take vitamin E and C on a daily basis because we think they can help to protect against some forms of cancer. More important, they can't hurt. Avoid exposure to potentially toxic chemicals in air, water and food. Don't smoke. Don't overdo exposure to the sun and the damaging effects of excess ultrviolet rays. Eat lots of fresh vegetables and fruits. Other than that, to use a well worn but appropriate phrase, "don't worry, be happy." Cancer will find you if you are destined to get it. Worrying about it won't protect you from getting sick, but it sure will take the fun out of life.

Fortunately, most people don't have cancer, even though at times it may seem that they do. Although many of us will develop some form of cancer during the course of life, many more people will suffer and die in this country from heart disease, stroke, gun shot wounds, domestic violence, auto accidents, and other preventable causes of death and suffering. In spite of this, we continue to fear the image of pain and suffering which is conjured up by that word-"cancer."

Talk to people who have experienced the diagnosis and treatment. You will get a very different story. While most will curse the discomfort they experienced and the side effects of the treatment programs, they will also tell you that the diagnosis made them a different person. As my wife has pointed out to me on a number of occasions, once you are told you have cancer, life is never the same again, but not always for the worse. Your view of the world changes and things that once seemed important lose significance. Forced to confront your own mortality, often earlier than expected, your values undergo a transformation. You learn to live for today and not be in fear of what tomorrow will bring, whether that means the next course of chemotherapy, the finding of a new metastases or recurrence, and other "what ifs".

Though cancer is indeed a terrible thing to have, it does not mean that life ends. It is not necessarily a death sentence. Your life has changed forever, but sometimes in a positive way. Many patients tell me that the diagnosis becomes a source of new strength. They learn to appreciate sights, sounds and smells they had previously taken for granted. They find positive things to say about people they formerly disliked and tend to overlook the countless frustrations which send us ordinary people into a dither. It is sad that most of us must be painfully forced to face catastrophic illness and mortality before we begin to appreciate the gift we have been given, but that is most typically the nature of our life today.

I often think of my many patients with cancer and the remarkable coping skills they teach me. Rather than retreat from the battle and hide away in their homes, many display an impressive commitment to carry on with life. I remember my dad, getting up from chemotherapy and driving five hours to a sales call in New Jersey in spite of nausea, weakness and painful mouth sores. When he called late that night from his motel room, his oncologist was struck by his determination. Even more impressive was his ability to present himself as positive and healthy and make a successful sale the next morning. I recall Sally, a strong and independent divorced woman in her 50's with metastatic breast cancer. She faced one procedure after another- chemotherapy, invasive attempts to open up her blocked bile ducts, bone marrow transplants, and repeated admissions to the hospital for infection. In spite of this, she maintained an astonishingly positive attitude. My visits and phone conversations are always received with her delightful sardonic wit. She managed to maintain her household, deal with her children's lifetime vicissitudes, and maintain an active schedule socializing with her friends and never (well, hardly ever) complained. There was Lawrence, a man of my own age who was felled by pancreatic cancer. To the very end, he remained a true gentleman, concerned most about his family and friends. In spite of his pain and apparent suffering, he always asked of a visitor about their own health and life situation.

The list is long and I could go on with dozens, perhaps even a few hundred examples of people who took their cancer in stride and either would not give in to self pity and fear, or who even gained from there illness and became stronger. It reminds me of a story my dad used to tell with great glee whenever I was feeling down or disheartened because things just weren't going my way. He told of the two young boys who came home to find they're bedrooms filled with horse manure. The parents came to the door of the first child and found him sitting at the edge of his room in tears. "Look at this mess. All my toys and pictures are ruined. I'll never clean this up." They consoled him and arranged for assistance to straighten things out. When they arrived at the door of the second son, however, they were astonished to find him shoveling away, throwing the refuse out the window and singing happily. Why, they asked was he so cheerful given his dismal lot? The boy replied with a smile and cheerful note to his voice (I still can picture my dad telling this part of the story), " With all this horse manure, there must be a pony in there somewhere!"

A politically powerful and highly successful businessman called me recently from an island in the Caribbean worried about what he thought might be blood in his urine. His concern, having just turned 50 was, of course, that this was a sign of cancer, perhaps of the prostate or the bladder. We talked at some length about the character of his urine discoloration, the absence of any additional symptoms and his general feeling of good health. It became quite clear to me that his urine color was not due to blood but rather a pigment from the large amounts of local island fruits and vegetables he had been eating. I reassured him and suggested that he stop in to the office after his return just to let me take a quick look at his urine under the microscope. His fear was relieved significantly. He noted that this was the first few days of vacation he had managed in the past 13 months, and he was feeling somewhat guilty about being away from his rather substantial responsibilities. Perhaps, I suggested, it was this sense of guilt which was in part driving his fear of suddenly finding some dread illness. We know each other well personally as well as professionally, so I felt comfortable saying to him, "Sam, don't wait for serious illness to learn that life is short and needs to be enjoyed as well as labored."

Cancer should not be the force that teaches us to appreciate the beauty and good fortune we have of waking up each day. We need to stop worrying about it, try our best to prevent it, treat it when needed, but not let the destructive forces of stress and fear manipulate our lives. Somewhere, in the midst of the troubles which beset us, there has to be a pony in there somewhere.

# *14*

## DEATH AND THE UNFORGIVING MINUTE

ndy was a bright, handsome promising high school senior who was a source of joy to his parents and siblings. Family and friends watched him mature slightly ahead of his peers into a thoughtful and caring young man who seemed to enjoy so many of the opportunities he faced. His life was changing from the challenges and frustrations of adolescence to wonderment at all that lay ahead. His interpretation of the world around him showed remarkable insight. Only recently, Andy's proud father, told me of his son's reading of "Zen and The Art of Motorcycle Repair." His mother adored him and he was his father's best friend. His dad loved to relate stories of the adventures they shared. I remember one story of the two of them going off on a short hike in the woods behind their ski house in New Hampshire. As they forged deeper into the hills, they soon found themselves totally lost. Without a compass and noting that one clump of trees or rocks looked like another, his dad was in a mild state of panic. He was able to calm himself with the confidence Andy had in his ability to find their way home. Several hours later, their "short hike" ended as they stumbled onto a trail that brought them back down the mountain. Adventures such as these tied the two closely together. Andy's dad glowed as he related similar tales and spoke proudly of his son's prospects for his upcoming college years.

Then the call came. His dad was covering for our group of doctors one Saturday morning when he was paged to a phone number which didn't seem familiar. It was the medical examiner in a community near Cape Cod who inquired if he was Andy's father. Anxiously replying in the affirmative, he was told that his son didn't survive the crash. Pale and near speechless, he inquired as to the nature of the call and soon found that his son, his only son, was lying dead at the local hospital, having been thrown from the back seat of a car in which he was sleeping as the driver fell asleep at the wheel. They were returning early from an after-prom party in order to be back in time to prepare for a test scheduled the next day. No alcohol and no dangerous road conditions were involved. The driver just got tired and went off the road. Now he was dead. Just like that.

Like so many unfortunate parents and families of young men and women killed on the highways, Andy's parents were bereft. Surely there was a mistake. This had to be somebody else's child. How can one find meaning in such a pointless and crushing death? If only he hadn't gone. If only the driver stayed awake. If only he was wearing his seatbelt. If only he had not been so determined to return to prepare for his exam. If only, if only, if only.... The shock soon led to tears and what seemed to be vain efforts to find solace and meaning in a life so full of promise cut off so young. Then Andy spoke to his family, friends and the world as if from the grave. Only a month earlier, his class had been involved in a discussion on the meaning of death after the tragic loss of a friend's parent. His comments at that time were so profound that a teacher recorded them in her class materials and wisely saw fit to bring them to the attention of Andy's parents on the day after his death.

"I am not afraid to die. I want it to be very peaceful and I will not want people to feel sorry for me; I just want them to remember me and rejoice in the days I was living."

I remember being deeply touched by the enormous wisdom of this young man when his dad showed me this quote on the evening after the funeral. Unlike our cultural obsession with dying and not getting enough toys before the end, Andy understood that life is about living, not dying. Don't grieve over the loss, he said. Think rather about the person he had been as a child, adolescent and young man. Remember him for his living and not for his dying. The words of this remarkable young man sent a clear message to all of us fortunate enough to have known him. So much of our issues about death are focused on the End and the Hereafter instead of on the Now and the present. Life is to be lived to the fullest, not frittered away worrying about death which will come in spite of our worry. Andy clearly got it right. He understood about filling the unforgiving minute.

Contrast Andy's story with that of Mary, a 94 year old woman with a sparkling personality who somehow lost her appreciation for the meaning of her life. Though nearly blind due to deterioration of the nerve cells in the back of her eyes and crippled by arthritis, she continued to live independently with the help of day care workers and some family. Mary had a ready smile and a quick wit. In spite of her difficulties, she expressed gratitude to any person who offered her the kindness of a helping hand. She barely ever complained about her physical limitations due to her heart failure and diabetes, and was ready to tell willing listeners how fortunate she felt to be alive on any given day.

Over the years she remained energetic and happy. In spite of this, I watched Mary's medical condition deteriorate and recognized the development of an ominous anemia in the presence of abnormal proteins in her blood. To me this meant that she was probably developing Multiple Myeloma, a disease of the bone marrow which could prove fatal if she did not succumb to some other illness first at her advanced age. I knew the treatment for this would be fraught with risks and offered no cure. Although treatment was available to suppress the abnormal cells in her bone marrow, I had nothing to offer this woman that would prolong her life. More important, she did not feel sick and she was unaware of any problems associated with the illness. Unfortunately, her eye doctor, a brilliant retina specialist, noted on a regular visit some changes in the back of the eye which raised his concern about possible blood diseases. He ordered some of the same tests I had performed regularly and told Mary that she had a blood problem and needed to speak to her medical doctor right away. When she anxiously called, I asked her to try to come in so we could discuss these test results.

Mary knew immediately where I was going with the diagnosis as I carefully explained the process in her bone marrow which was crowding out healthy cells and causing the changes which were seen in her eyes.

"Do I have cancer?" She was straight-forward in her question and wanted a direct response. Yes, I said, this is a form of cancer.

"Then I'm going to die?" This was more an anxious question than a statement of an obvious fact. I was startled by her response and had to collect my thoughts for a moment. I wanted to say of course you're going to die. You're 94 years old and this is the time when people die. Rather than hit her over the head with this painful truth, I needed to better understand her reaction to what I had just told her. I asked her what she feared about the diagnosis of cancer, expecting to hear about pain, suffering from treatments and loss of independence.

Instead, she said "I don't want to die. I'm not ready for it."

I couldn't stop myself from responding with what must have been a tone of incredulity, "But you're 94. We all are going to die."

"Not me. Not yet. There's a woman in my building who just turned 100. I want to be around at least that long. You've kept me well until now (I knew this to be a painful misperception on her part.) You'll keep me going until then." This was stated with such force and certainty, that it startled me. I knew what lay ahead for her if we opted for treatment and was hesitant to recommend that she choose such an option. In spite of her strong will to live, she was medically quite fragile. As I began to explain the options for treatment, she insisted that we get started. I explained that a bone marrow test would be necessary to confirm the diagnosis before we began any treatment.

"Won't that be painful? I don't want any pain."

I explained that while the test was simple and involved only momentary discomfort, there would be some slight pain. I tried to explain the mild and evanescent character of the pain associated with this procedure, knowing full well that this was the least of her problems should we decide to go ahead with treatment.

"Why can't you just give me some medicine for this? Why should I have to suffer through tests? Can't you just give me a pill or something? You're a smart doctor."

I recognized her ambivalence. She didn't want to die, but she didn't want to suffer either. Who could fault such an attitude. On the other hand, I had to decide about giving her medication to treat the condition which, in her frail condition could cause more illness, suffering and even death. How was I to present this to her without destroying her hope and joy in life? I explained that I could only treat her problem if I could prove the diagnosis with the test. There would be too much risk involved in the treatment without knowing this with certainty. She relented and agreed to the bone marrow test and then embarked on a course of very weak simple oral chemotherapy which she should have tolerated. The dose of the medication is calculated based on the size and age of a patient as well as factors controlling handling of the drug by the body's metabolic functions. The dose should have been correct. Instead, within a month Mary's white blood count had plummeted so low that she required hospitalization for a week to recover from severe infection and 5 weeks to recover in a rehabilitation hospital. She now struggles from week to week to attend visits at the oncology clinic where she has blood extracted and medicine injected.

Mary's life has become focused on beating back death. She has no time to fill any unforgiving minutes. Quality has been exchanged for quantity. Each time I see her now, weaker and struggling for each step and each breath, I wonder to myself, In this frail, wonderful 94 year old woman, did I do right to offer her medication? Perhaps I should have said, "I'm sorry Mary. We have no reasonable safe treatment to offer you. In spite of that, you feel OK and seem to be managing as well as usual. Let us instead focus on making your remaining days as comfortable and fulfilling as possible."

Mary, like most people in our culture, believed in the power of modern medicine above the absolute nature of the life cycle. Was I wrong to allow her to exercise that belief? Clearly, our culture supports the need to provide medical treatment in this setting. Others do not. As a society, we need to address this issue squarely. Should we promote prolongation of life as our greatest goal? Given the promises we make to cure illness and the miracles in store for us with genetic engineering, this question will become increasingly important not only to physicians, but to society as a whole. Can we afford to focus and improve both quality and quantity of life simultaneously?

Patients like Mel helped me to focus on the issue of quality versus quantity. At 80 years of age he considered himself fit and healthy. He saved any medically related complaints for the once a year visit to my office. Even those were elicited only on intensive questioning. He ached here and there, occasionally felt a little tired, and his urine stream had slowed. "What do you expect at my age? I'm fine. Everything is OK," he would say. Rather than a time for concern, his medical visits were more a peremptory exercise which he performed out of deference to his three physician children. Indeed, he always appeared trim and fit, an example of perfect health. He exercised regularly, ate a Spartan diet and his physical conditioning was remarkable. With the exception of rather striking baldness, his physical examination, electrocardiogram and blood tests, as well as the usual screening tests were consistently normal. His business ventures had been successful, yet he lived a simple and unpretentious style. His energy at this point in life was focused on assisting his children, winding up his business interests, and playing golf.

I was surprised when I was interrupted while examining a patient late on a Thursday afternoon by an urgent call from Mel's daughter who was on her way to an emergency room near her Dad's golf course. He was taken by ambulance from the 18th hole, having collapsed after finishing a round. I reassured her that I would get right on the matter and dialed ahead to the hospital. I learned from the emergency room doctor that Mel had suffered a stroke. He appeared comfortable but not terribly alert. We soon found that his stroke was massive with extensive hemorrhage (bleeding) inside the brain. The pressure this created on the brain and the loss of brain function due to all the damaged tissue caused him to become progressively less alert and unresponsive. We watched him slowly slip away from us. Mel had previously made his wishes clear to his family that he would never accept a life of dependency or infirmity. Life supports and rehabilitation were never an issue. He was kept comfortable and quiet in the intensive care unit. Within a few hours he fell into a deep coma never to regain consciousness and died with his family at his side in the intensive care unit less than 6 hours after collapsing on the golf course.

When I met with his children, they were obviously shattered by the loss of this man whom they loved and on whom they were so dependent as a source of guidance and strength. At the same time, they commented on what a full and satisfying life he led. He never had a day of illness or suffering, and "shot his age" of 80 on the golf course, a life-long goal. He never feared death, and never allowed concern over it's inevitability to enter into his plans or activities. His greatest concern was the care and support of his wife after his death. Mel went through life with no demonstrable fear of mortality and exited on terms he could hardly have negotiated better had he the opportunity. While a few more years would have been nice, perhaps to see one of his grandchildren graduate from college, he knew that he had no guarantees. He was unwilling to accept the inevitable disability and dependency that was certain to be waiting in the years ahead.

It would appear that Mel died a near perfect death made easier by his clearly expressed feelings about life, death and medical intervention. And yet, the problems that followed reminded me that the tragedy of death is often more for those who are left behind, not so much for the deceased. Mel's fears for his wife were well founded. Her dependency and passive nature during his life turned into a severe depression complicated by progressive confusion. The strength, guidance and support of his personality and presence are now gone. When she comes to see me now with her attendants, she tearfully mourns his loss and is unable to move ahead emotionally. While Mel understood the unforgiving minute, his widow doesn't even know there is a clock.

Mel's death was easier and natural largely because of his open discussion about his wishes and his clearly expressed view of life. Unfortunately today this is more the exception than the rule. The absence of such guidelines either informally or in the form of a living will creates an ethical and clinical mess about end of life decisions. In my earlier days in practice, before managed care made me a slave to paperwork and regulations, I had time to make weekly rounds at a nursing home not far from my office. I recall vividly one warm and sunny afternoon standing in a room as I looked across the bed at a mute and wasted old man. The pale yellow walls contrasted with the white sheet neatly drawn up to his neck. The air was filled with the pungent odor of dried urine. In the background I could hear the sound of some other less sedated patient calling out a monosyllabic noise. Otherwise there was only silence.

I knew this man and I knew that an elderly relative came to visit him and sit by his bedside for a few brief minutes once or twice a week. The remainder of the time he spent in exactly this position or propped up in a chair in the main room on the second floor of this building. Three times a day an aid entered the room and placed food in his mouth and waited for him to silently gum the food and swallow it down. His sheets and clothing were changed once and sometimes twice a day if needed and his skin was carefully protected with rubbing, creams, powders and body repositioning. There he would sit or lie in silence except for the noises of other more active patients or the radio which I often found blaring at his bedside to a station which I knew had to be the choice of the nurses or aides. No octogenarian I know would ever have selected the sounds coming from the little electronic box.

Such was his existence, if it could be called that. I had no authority to discontinue his care or to allow him to die a natural death. No effort was made when he was more alive to determine his wishes as to how this was to be handled. If he stopped breathing or some other emergency arose, I was compelled to send him to the hospital and treat him until the time when nature took its course.

On that particular day, as I gazed through the curtained window beside his bed, I saw the park across the street where a young mother pushed a carriage along a neatly trimmed path. She stopped to bend down and tuck in the white and pink blanket around her baby. They passed by a bench where an elderly woman sat quietly staring at the pigeons which converged on the crumbs she had cast on the ground. The foliage was green and soft and a gentle spring breeze passed through the tall birch trees revealing the alternating dark and light shade on either side of the leaves. I paused to wonder at the juxtaposition of these life experiences in my visual field. I can still hear myself thinking "Which is reality here? Which of these images is the life that I trained to maintain and support?" By helping to preserve this shadow of a human being, am I really helping life or denying death. Whose values am I maintaining by preventing this man from following life's natural cycles? How are we to die in this culture of technology and denial of death?

As I have confronted the question of life and death for my patients and my family over the past 25 years of my medical career, this moment has returned to me repeatedly. We all will experience death in our loved ones and ultimately in ourselves Because of this, we all need some moral and ethical construct to help us cope with the inevitability of the dying process, unless we are denied the opportunity by death's occasional precipitous swiftness and unpredictability. We need some map to help us find the way to resolve the conflict between the force which drives us to fight to live and the realization that we must at some point give up the fight and accept the finality of our existence.

An unpleasant experience with a family who were unwilling to accept death at any cost brought this question into clear focus for me. Recent immigrants to this country who believed that they were now able to receive the best medical care in the world, they demanded maximal care for their ailing mother for every problem which arose. She was unresponsive and unable to communicate, dependent on feedings through tubes and intravenous fluid and completely incontinent of bowel and bladder function. In essence, she was in a vegetative state. There was no prospect of her ever recovering. In spite of this, she was repeatedly transferred from her nursing home bed to the hospital emergency room and intensive care unit.

How can we all acquire the wisdom and foresight of Andy or Mel? Too many times I have watched or participated in the emotional and intellectual conflict surrounding end of life decisions. Living wills and the discussions they create are a new and important tool for dealing with this.

On several occasions, when her heart stopped or she developed a decrease in her breathing capacity, she underwent cardiac resuscitation with pounding and compression of her frail chest along with the passage of a large tube down her throat into her windpipe. Catheters were passed into her bladder and tubes were pushed up her rectum. Needles were stuck into her arms, neck, spine and chest on various occasions. Watching and ordering these procedures had become a painful process for me. I tried repeatedly to discuss the possibility of terminating her care with her family. They were adamantly opposed to any interruption of care and made clear their goal of keeping her alive as long as possible.

I began to see my treatment of this woman as a form of torture for both of us. She was subjected to what I knew to be painful treatments because of her family's unwillingness to let her die in peace. I was forced to inflict this treatment in what I came to see as an inhumane effort. Each time I visited her at the nursing home, I would stand at her bedside as I did with the nursing home patient mentioned earlier and wonder about my role as physician. I found it easier to answer the question this time. This was not the life I had trained to help and support. I tried to address this issue of quality vs. quantity of life with her son and daughter. They remained adamant. I finally told them that, if they were insistent on maintaining their plan of treatment, I could not in good conscience continue to be the caregiver for their mother. I offered to find another doctor for them. They were understandably angry since they did not appreciate my point of view. I was fired. I watched her return to the hospital under the care of another physician on several occasions over the next few months until she finally died at the age of 87 in the intensive care unit receiving the best modem science had to offer.

This experience did not leave me feeling vindicated or in any way satisfied. I felt as if I had failed the patient by allowing her to suffer and her family by not helping them to understand the futility and self-serving nature of their efforts. They all came to this country expecting the best of everything. Our medical system promised them that, but allowed the issue of best quality to be confused with greatest quantity. For this reason as well as what I suspect were some cultural differences, the patient's family members were unwilling to cope with the important change from a determined battle for life to acceptance of the inevitability of death.

People who manage this transition better than others find death less of an enemy in battle. I watched my father deal with this in the last weeks of his life. For seven years he fought a stubborn war against his lymphoma, refusing to surrender his frenetic existence as a salesman par excellence. He would rise from his chemotherapy treatments to rush off to a sales call with no inhibitions about his loss of hair or diminished physical stature. Those he called on will report to this day that even at his weakest, he was the most determined and effective salesman they knew. His motto was never give up, never give in. Hard work, he was fond of saying, never killed anybody. This applied to both an unrelenting customer as well as a tenacious cancer. Whether you wanted his product or not, as a buyer, you had to admire his pluck and courage.

The one exception to my father's work ethic was fishing. He could go fishing anytime and sit for hours without a bite as his boat gently rocked at anchor. I can't think of anything that gave him more pleasure with the possible exception of visits from one of his 15 grandchildren. If he could combine the two, so much the better. I remember each year of the last few as I accompanied him to put the boat away for the season how sad I felt that this would be his last. Yet he rallied again and again each season to get back out to his favorite spots off Boston Harbor. I could never bring myself to join him on these trips because I couldn't tolerate the endless sitting at anchor and dragging fish to the surface to suffocate them in a barrel. I think it was one of his great disappointments, and certainly mine, that I never joined him in this pursuit. Sadly, I thought it was just about fishing.

After trying every treatment option available and investigating those that were not, my father realized that the end was imminent. He was in constant pain and his breathing was hard. I remember the visit from Dr. Schnipper, his oncologist, as he gently in his soft, kindly voice gave the bad news. Tumor growths had sprouted on his skin and in his essential organs. He told my dad that they had tried everything, and he had to face the truth. There was nothing left. It was hard to believe that only a few weeks earlier he was busy making sales calls on the phone. I believe this was one of the most difficult moments in his life. He called me to his bedside and took my hand. In the weak voice he had remaining he asked me if I would see him as a quitter if he surrendered to his illness. Fighting back the tears, I told him that nobody would ever call Al Solomon a quitter. It was time to take the short odds and play the hand you were dealt.

In his remaining days we managed to gather most of the family around to celebrate my parents' fiftieth anniversary. He took time to speak privately with each one of his children to leave an individual message. Dad always had a way of making each of us feel we were the special child. My mother was at his side constantly. When he finally stopped breathing early in the morning two weeks later, he went knowing he had spent his time well and satisfied that although he had nothing of material value to leave to his family, he left behind a legacy of values and standards for his descendants to follow. It was only after his death that I realized the trips out into the harbor on his boat were not just about fishing or wasting time. They were about quality of life. Fishing was my father's way of stopping to smell the roses. I missed my opportunity to share this with him, probably my greatest regret in life. But I learned the lesson well. Quality of life is more important by far than quantity.

During a synagogue service in my home-town on the Jewish New Year, one of our rabbis, Joshua Elkin, spoke on the complexities of dealing with the end of life.

"I have sat with many people who knew that they were dying. I have held their hands and tried to ease the passage for them. What they taught me is that people are not afraid of dying; they are afraid of not having lived."

Instead of worrying away our days over the fear of dying, we need to remember the unforgiving minute. We need to heed Andy's advice and rejoice in living.

# *15*

## JUST WHAT THE DOCTOR ORDERED

Traditional western medicine trains physicians to ferret out rare and unusual disorders. We have become increasingly skilled at treating these as well as managing more serious illnesses. We are not particularly good, however, at preventing those medical issues around which much fear is generated. Nor are the non-traditional alternative sources of care, for that matter. While we try in many ways, we cannot prevent leukemia, lung cancer, heart disease, stroke, diabetes, colitis and ileitis, multiple sclerosis, brain tumors, skin cancers, cirrhosis and many other illnesses. But you can have an impact on many of these.

While my message to this point has been to avoid worrying about your health, there is much you can do to assure the best chance for a long and productive life. Living healthy is mostly your responsibility. You own this job and should pursue it to the best of your ability. Your health care provider is like a safari guide whose job it is to keep you on the straight and narrow path through the jungle of life, watch out for hazards and deal with avoidable and unavoidable problems along the way. If you stray into dangerous areas on your own or unintentionally, your doctor-guide will often have to rescue you using all the wisdom, skill, science and technology available.

This may sound like a contradiction. Don't worry, be happy. Take responsibility, be vigilant. Let's look at it differently. If you are fortunate enough to learn to play the piano at an early age, you know that you need to keep playing to maintain your skills. You may play an hour a day or twice a week, but you don't obsess about playing all the time. The skill is learned and intact. In the same manner, once you have learned the skills and techniques to lead a healthy life, you may need to think about it once or twice a day, but you don't need to worry all the time. And just as you will not likely ever play like Artur Rubenstein, you may also never achieve perfect health. In either case, if the genes aren't right you can waste your life worrying about what you can't achieve.

So let's cut to the chase. What follows may seem sometimes overly simplistic and other times preachy, but it is the truth. Take it or leave it. It's your choice.

## WHAT YOU NEED TO DO FOR YOUR HEALTH

**1. Don't use tobacco.**—Using tobacco is just plain dumb. I grant there are tremendous social pressures to smoke cigarettes or cigars, chew tobacco or suck on a pipe. More important, nicotine is a potent addictive agent which has been used by the tobacco industry to foster dependence. Quitting is hard. I know. I did it in college. Still there is help available in the form of support groups, nicotine supplements and medication. Some patients worry about the side effects of the various treatments. As far as I can tell, there is nothing we can give you to help stop smoking that is more dangerous than continued smoking, short of putting you in front of a firing squad. Just in case you're unclear of the reasons for not smoking, let me go through the risks.

Smoking causes cancer. Not just lung cancer, but also cancer of the nose, throat, mouth, larynx, esophagus, stomach, bladder and probably colon. There is an association as well with cancer of the pancreas, breast and probably others I can't think of right now. It also causes heart disease, aneurysms, vascular disease leading to loss of circulation to the legs, and stroke. It causes poor pregnancy outcome. It damages the lungs leading to chronic bronchitis, emphysema and respiratory failure. Menopause usually comes earlier. From a cosmetic point of view, it leads to a hoarse voice from damaged vocal cords, shortened posture with advancing age, thinning and wasting of the jawbone with accelerated loss of teeth and wrinkled skin. Because of its effects on small blood vessels, it probably contributes to impotence. It's also dirty, discolors the skin and makes you smell of tobacco.

Given all this, why would anybody start smoking? If already smoking, why would anybody continue? Smoking cigarettes is the equivalent of stepping out onto the highway in front of an 18-wheeler over and over again. If you choose to take this step, be prepared for the consequences. If you want to get out of harm's way, there is help available. It's your choice.

**2. Don't drink alcohol to excess.**- This has become a tough issue. New studies indicate that some people have improved cholesterol patterns, with 1-2 glasses of alcohol each day. The liquor industry has jumped at this opportunity to promote good health through the grape. Like most issues in life, however, it's not that simple. While some people benefit from the salutory effects of alcohol on cholesterol, many do not. In fact, only a select group of people with a particular cholesterol pattern in their blood will have a positive result from the daily intake of alcohol. Others will develop a substantial worsening of their cholesterol and other blood fat levels. For some people with a genetic predisposition or serious personal problems, one or two drinks may lead to alcoholism.

The uncontrolled consumption of alcohol is one of the most damaging forces in our culture today. Aside from effects on individual health it can worsen job performance, lead to interpersonal conflict and domestic strife and cause careless and irresponsible activities leading to injury and often death to others. For many, the problem begins in the teenage years with binge drinking on weekends as a rite of adolescent rebellion. By the time high school is over drinking may have progressed to "a few beers with dinner." I am struck by the number of 22 to 30 year old men I see who consume up to a case of beer a week, clearly an excessive amount. Even if the behavior is denied, a medical evaluation often points to the problem with the finding of elevated blood pressure, heart abnormalities, abnormal levels of liver enzymes in the blood, excess fat floating in the blood stream and abnormal numbers and shapes of blood cells.

Often patients will come in quite proud of their consumption of red wine, initiated purely to prolong their life. If this use of alcohol is based on medicinal reasons, knowledge of the impact of alcohol on your health is important. Daily intake of even small amounts of alcohol can lead to diabetes and liver problems. Some studies suggest that regular alcohol increases the risk of osteoporosis and breast cancer. In vulnerable patients, even small amounts of alcohol can trigger heart rhythm abnormalities, brain injury or other neurologic problems. Don't assume safety with alcohol use simply because you heard it on the news or read it in some magazine. A medical evaluation and laboratory tests can give you some information as to how alcohol will affect your body. Unfortunately, some of the effects of alcohol are silent and cannot be predicted.

While I am not opposed to alcohol use and enjoy a glass of good wine with a fine meal or a cocktail with friends at a social event, I am aware of the potential effect it might have on my body and I choose to have a drink in spite of this. Alcohol is not inherently evil. Rather your ability to control consumption and recognize side effects determines safety. If you understand the potential risks and benefits, you can make a reasonable decision. It's your choice.

**3. Try to exercise a little each day.**- Remember the words of Satchel Paige to "jangle things around to keep the juices flowing." We were not created to be sedentary. The enormous and powerful muscles of our lower back, thighs and legs were designed for more than sitting on the sofa, sitting at a desk or stepping on the accelerator. Even if we attribute all of our body characteristics to evolution, the tremendous reserve capacity of the heart and lungs did not develop for hyperventilation at the site of a movie star or for gesticulation and shouting over a touch down scored on television. We neglect the use of these marvelous body components at our own peril. It's like owning an automobile with 400 horsepower and using it only to drive around the corner to the mall. After a while the spark plugs gum up, the gas peddle sticks and the tire treads start to disintegrate. When you need the power it won't be there. While some can vegetatively survive into advanced age without breaking a sweat, those who I have seen remain sharp and agile and able to enjoy life remain physically and mentally active well into their later years.

Some take this message to exercise as motivation to achieve supreme conditioning in the form of marathon running, triathalon training, long distance bicycling and the like. These people should be admired for their determination and commitment. For the rest of us, achievable goals are more reasonable. Most of us have substantial demands on time and energy at home, at work or in our community. Two or three hours a day of fitness training is not an option. On the other hand, we miss many opportunities in the course of the day to pump up our muscles, lungs and cardiovascular system. We need to use our physical abilities instead of fossil fuel powered machinery whenever possible. This means take the stairs and not the escalator or elevator whenever possible. During the great oil crisis two decades ago, signs at elevators appeared all over the country which said, "You'll save energy and the environment too if you'll walk up one and walk down two." Go back to using the stairs.

Try walking at least a little each day. Twenty to thirty minutes of brisk walking, particularly in the early morning, helps to pump up the cardiovascular system. If you can't find the time for planned walking, fit it into your normal activities like walking to the train or walking at lunch time. Use common sense when and where to walk. Don't walk outside when the weatherman reports conditions to be unhealthful. Don't walk in areas known to be dangerous. Whenever possible, walk with one or more friends. Be sure to dress appropriately. Don't overdress with bulky heavy clothing when not necessary. Use comfortable synthetic soled supportive footwear. Keep your arms moving when you walk to stimulate your upper body and to keep blood circulating from your hands back to your heart. Take the time to enjoy the world around as you walk. If you don't stop to smell the flowers, at least exercise your eyes and your soul with the beauty of a new sunrise or sunset, new buds on tree branches, spring flowers, the changing color of trees in the fall. Exercise your face with a smile and hello to passers by. A good walk can change your outlook on the whole world.

Walking is not always an option. In these circumstances, all sorts of possibilities are available. You can join a gym if you can make the time commitment. The local Y and other organizations usually have facilities and programs scheduled at convenient times. If this doesn't work for you, then get a piece of home equipment which you will use. Don't spend $1200 for a treadmill if you're just going to throw clothing over it. Be sure to try different types of machines at your local retail store or at a friend's house. Look for used equipment in the local newspaper or pennysaver.

Sometimes exercise just isn't possible. Weather, work, meetings, child-care and countless other responsibilities intervene. Even though you're committed to regular exercise, you slip off for a few days a week or even longer. Don't feel guilty or ashamed. Life is what it is. You do the best you can. On the other hand, whenever possible try to find some time. The most difficult time in any exercise program is the last 5 minutes before you go out the door or get on your machine. That's when you can think of at least a half dozen reasons not to exercise that day. Push past these feelings. To steal a hot current marketing phrase, just do it. It's your choice.

**4. Eat Sensibly.**- Eating is such a natural function, you would think we could do it without screwing things up so badly. Unfortunately, our culture is overloaded with easily available low quality, high fat, high caloric content food. We tend to load ourselves up with foods derived from animal fats and relatively low in natural vitamins. The average person can look at what he eats at each meal and easily recognize the good, the bad and the ugly. Just because a given food is habit, like pizza or fast food hamburgers, doesn't mean they're healthy. It takes a break from nationalistic fervor to accept the truth that bacon, eggs and home fries for breakfast, a cheeseburger and fries for lunch and steak with bread and potatoes for supper is just not healthful.

Where do you begin? First of all, it is clear we need to reduce our intake of foods derived from animals. The risks of heart disease, colon cancer and probably breast cancer are all increased in proportion to the amount consumed from these sources. Although animal meat is an important source of protein, some essential amino acids and vitamins, these can also come from grains, legumes and fish. Once the issues of environmental management needed to produce these other sources in large enough volume can be overcome there will be little excuse for avoiding these healthier sources of protein and vitamins.

Fruits and vegetables are another area where we neglect ourselves. The latest dietary recommendations from the American Dietetic Association (ADA) and the Food and Drug Administration (FDA) suggest 3-5 servings of vegetables and 2-4 servings of fruit each day. Compared to the normal American diet, that's a lot.

Much has been learned about nutritional needs. It seems that a lot of what we were taught as children was wrong. We need to rethink our approach to food. The essential elements of the new healthy diet are in general, eat less, eat less meat and more grains, eat more vegetables and fruits, avoid sweets and fatty foods and try to eat fish at least a couple of times a week. Try to eat foods not contaminated with chemicals, a most difficult task in our mass marketing culture. Nobody has proven scientifically that eating foods produced organically (that is without artificial chemicals) is safer and healthier. It's just one of those things that intuitively makes sense. Still there are no guarantees of safety. As Dr. Andrew Weil points out in Healthy Living, many foods, whether organic or not, can be harmful. For example, I was surprised to learn that uncooked white mushrooms, widely available at salad bars, may contain naturally occurring cancer causing substances. And who would have suspected that sprouts, the epitome of the crunchy, healthy diet, are a potential source of infection from Salmonella bacteria?

Patients often ask for a place to read about food and diets. The information is more manageable if you can see it in print. Several good books are available. The latest which I find appealing is Dieting for Dummies by Jane Kirby. Probably the best source for such information is the ADA's website at www.eatright.org. The American Heart Association has excellent diet and cookbooks available by contacting their local office. For those who want to understand more about what is wrong with the way America eats I recommend Diet for a New America by H. J. Kramer.

Most of us can do a better job of deciding what we eat. The process can be as simple as dropping the cream in our morning coffee in exchange for 1% or even skim milk. Avoid the usual high animal fat lunch and supper normal for most of us and substitute grains, vegetable, pasta and rice. You can attempt a more in depth effort to reconstruct and redesign the way you eat using written sources and dietitians as guides. In either case, eating healthier can be done. Whether you maintain your current style or choose to change will alter your health and sense of well-being. It's your choice.

5. Use common sense.- Learn to approach illness the way our grandparents did. Don't rush off to call the doctor without giving some thought to the source and nature of your complaints. Remember that we are often the victims of our own foolishness. If you know what caused the problem, try to approach it logically. Be patient and allow your body to heal. Following a few simple rules can avoid unnecessary, expensive and sometimes risky treatments.

If you develop muscle or joint pain, try to remember how it happened. Lifting, pushing, pulling, carrying objects beyond normal ability will frequently lead to pain. Bending or leaning in one position for a prolonged time can trigger muscle spasms. Sudden forced movements or trivial bumps can present with terrible pain a few days later. In the first 24 hours after an injury apply ice to reduce swelling. If possible, try to rest the area involved. After that first day, begin to apply heat for 15-30 minutes at a time. Warm is better than hot. After the first two to three days things should be improving. This leads to one of the most important common sense rules: Good things get better. Bad things get worse. If you're improving steadily, be patient. If not, call your doctor.

When it comes to colds and respiratory infections, try to recognize your illness by the company it keeps. If everybody at work, at home or at school has the same annoying runny nose, scratchy throat, head congestion and cough and they all seem to be surviving, don't rush to the doctor if you have the same. Remember a cold is a cold is a cold-usually. The average virus cold will last from 5 to 10 days. On the other hand, if your symptoms are debilitating, if your temperature persists for more than 48 to 72 hours, it's time to call the doctor. Also, if your cold seems to be going away but fever returns or develops new after 6 or 7 days, call the doctor. At anytime during your illness if your fever continues to rise, if you become short of breath or develop sinus or chest pain, call your doctor. Watch for anything unusual in other bodily functions such as a rash, a swollen joint, a change in urine appearance. Don't hesitate to call if you're not sure.

Gastrointestinal symptoms follow a different pattern. Except for seasonal viral gastroenteritis with nausea, vomiting and diarrhea which tends to occur in community wide outbreaks in the spring and fall., most acute gastrointestinal symptoms are self inflicted. If you overeat, particularly highly spiced or seasoned foods, don't be surprised if you experience nausea, distress, belching or cramps. If you know some specific foods tend to upset you such as wine, dairy products, Chinese or Italian food, pepperoni pizza or chocolate eclairs, don't rush to call the doctor when the symptoms hit. Use whatever worked before. Learn to try antacids. Liquids work faster. Tablets containing calcium last longer. On the other hand, if you are experiencing indigestion with almost every meal or your symptoms are continuous for more than 2 weeks, then it's time to get medical attention.

Constipation and diarrhea are important symptoms if they represent a prolonged change in bowel function. Consider first whether this change was precipitated by something new. Did you start a new medication which might change your bowel habit? Check this out with your pharmacist. Did you recently change your diet? For many people, foods like rice and some herbal teas are terribly constipating. If you regularly consume high fiber foods like whole wheat breads and bran cereals or muffins, a change in intake can lead to abrupt onset of constipation. If your bowel function returns to normal with a simple readjustment in your diet, there is no need to seek immediate medical attention.

Of course, you always have the option to see your doctor if you feel unsure or find your symptoms too frightening to manage on your own. Don' t be ashamed or afraid to seek medical help. On the other hand, try to allow a little time to see if the problem will resolve on its own so long as it is improving. When your routine is disrupted by the sudden onset of new symptoms you can give it some thought or you can seek immediate medical attention. Unless the problem seems to imminently threaten life or limb, it makes sense to wait a little and see what happens.  In either case, it's your choice.

**6. Get proper medical care.**- Whether you choose to see an MD, an osteopath or a nurse practitioner, follow several important rules.  If you are a woman and are sexually active, you need to be seen annually starting in your late teens.  If you are celibate or having a pause in sexual activity, then every two years until age 40 is reasonable. Men who are in good health with no active medical problems should have a general exam every two to three years until age 40.  In spite of all the debate about frequency of examinations, I believe strongly that everybody should be seen once a year over 40.  An annual visit to the doctor is more than simply a mechanical process of examining different parts of the body.  The annual visit if done properly is a reality check-time to remember your mortality to think about issues such as lifestyle, smoking, alcohol use, exercise, family and job stress. For many people, it is the only time in the course of the year when somebody says, "How do you feel? Is everything OK at home?" and actually pays attention to your response.

In order to accomplish this goal you need to find a care provider who is not only eminently qualified to assess and treat your medical issues, but knows how to ask the right questions and will listen to the answer.  This doesn't mean a 15 or 20 minute visit when you come in for a sore elbow or a virus cold. It does mean that when the chips are down, in the setting of a devastating illness or enormous personal stress, your doctor is ready to listen, guide and support.

Proper medical care means more than listening.  It also means regular monitoring of essential body systems by reviewing historical patterns, a careful examination and regularly scheduled prophylactic treatments and  screening tests.  A limited list would include:

Hepatitis B vaccine in young adults
Diphtheria-Tetanus toxoid every 10 years
Hepatitis A vaccine in travelers
Influenza and Pneumonia vaccine in high risk patients and those
    over 65
Regular PAP smears

Mammograms

Flexible sigmoidoscopy or colonoscopy every 5 years after age
50

Prostate exam and PSA test where indicated

If you have followed all these guidelines and still feel unsure about your health, get another opinion. A good doctor who is confident in his or her skills will never object to this option even though it may represent a slight blow to the ego. If you trust your doctor, simply say you're not leaving his care. You'd just like to have things confirmed or have a fresh opinion. Make that clear with the next doctor you see. You don't want everything repeated. You just want another experienced professional to listen to the story, review the facts and give an honest judgment. Then go back to your regular doctor.

These procedures, regular checkups, immunizations, screening tests are recommendations, not absolute rules. Whether or not you follow through as advised is your decision. If you don't, you may be fortunate and still avoid preventable illness and disease. On the other hand, neglecting these recommendations could lead to disastrous consequences such as stroke, heart attack or kidney failure from untreated hypertension. Regular stool blood exams, breast exams, mammography and sigmoidoscopy are our current best method for preventing or eliminating potentially fatal cancers. Wear your seatbelt when in cars and helmets when bicycling.

See your doctor regularly and do the proper tests and you will increase your likelihood of surviving longer and healthier. Or you can take your chances. It's your choice.

**7. Find some joy and meaning in life.**- If you hate your job, your family life is a mess, the pressures of finances are overwhelming or you are burdened with sadness, you will feel unwell.

Those who deal with these issues know the painful error of the statement, "If you have your health, you have everything." Somehow you have to find your way to wake up grateful for a new day. It matters little what you eat or how much you exercise if you can't appreciate each day. Many of the world's great religions begin each day with a prayer of thanks for awakening. There must be some reason for such a universal understanding of the gift of a new day.

We are all so busy with our responsibilities, it is often too late before we realize how much time we have lost. We should not have to wait for the reality of Nabokov's hangman's noose to focus our minds on what really matters. Certainly it is useless and non-productive to live in fear of matters over which you have no control. At the same time, it may be hard to find the pony in the manure life throws your way.

If you can't find a clear path on your own, help is available. Speak to your doctor or your clergyman. Both can help you independently or in concert. Whether through counseling, medication, religious rededication or some combination of the three, you can find some joy in life. Health without happiness has no meaning or value.

## CONCLUSION

Though I don't demand a change in behavior on the part of my patients, I encourage them to recognize that all these issues are areas where they can improve their likelihood of living a long and fruitful life. Sure, there are no guarantees. Sure you can be killed tomorrow by some freak accident. I am often told by those wishing to deny their role in managing health, you can be hit by a car while crossing the street. While I acknowledge the truth inherent in such a statement, I like to point out that such an event is less likely if you look both ways beforehand. In the same manner, if you approach your health with your eyes open, looking "both ways" can reduce your risk of unexpected disaster.

All of these issues reviewed are potential pitfalls. You can worry about medical problems all day long. Radio, television, newspapers, and now the internet bombard us with new diseases to fear, new treatments to try or tests to have performed. You can count your vitamins in the morning, your calories consumed during the day and burned up with exercise. You can live in fear of every burp, belch, sneeze, cough, ache or strain. You can hide from the sun and live in fear of chemical contamination. You can look at yourself in the mirror each day and assess the amount to of fat needed to be shed.

On the other hand, life is short. There is so much to do and so little time in which to do it. Rather than obsess, you can choose to recognize that life is about so much more than worrying about your health. It is not about being a perfect patient or perfect physical specimen. It is certainly not about living forever. The secret to living well before we face the hangman's noose is to accept our own mortality, to exercise proper caution, to avoid obsessive behavior towards our health and avoid the distractions which prevent us from enjoying life.

Follow the few simple rules:

1. Don't use tobacco
2. Don't drink to excess
3. Try to exercise a little each day
4. Eat sensibly
5. Use common sense when you don't feel well
6. Get proper medical care
7. Find some joy and meaning in life

Do the best you can. If you fall short or fail to meet your goals, don't fret or obsess. You may decide to ignore all the suggestions. That's OK as long as you're willing to take your chances and accept the consequences. Doing what's best is not very hard. It's your choice.

Just remember, don't worry and be healthy.